Homoeopathy

FOR BABIES & CHILDREN

A P

Beth MacEoin

Headway · Hodder & Stoughton

British Library Cataloguing in Publication Data

MacEoin, Beth
  Homoeopathy for Babies and Children:
  Parent's Guide
  I. Title
  615.532

ISBN 0 340 60906 0

First published 1994
Impression number 10 9 8 7 6 5 4 3 2 1
Year   1999 1998 1997 1996 1995 1994

Typeset by Wearset, Boldon, Tyne and Wear.
Printed in Great Britain for Hodder & Stoughton Educational, a division of Hodder Headline Plc, 338 Euston Road, London NW1 3BH by Cox & Wyman Ltd, Reading

This book is dedicated to the memory of Sammy

CONTENTS

Foreword

Why is there a growing demand and interest in alternative and complementary forms of medicine and therapy from the public, government and the medical professions?

Firstly, there is an increasing awareness among consumers that orthodox treatments can also *cause* illness, from the side-effects of drugs and from dependency. Many people often feel deprived of a sense of self, being excluded from the decision-making process about their treatment. Their bodies are treated as machine parts rather than as a whole, and many seek alternative, holistic treatment as a way of taking responsibility for their own, and their family's, health.

From the government and medical establishment, perhaps it is concern over the costs of modern medicine, which are alarmingly high, due to expensive equipment and modern technology. The health service seems to generate an ever-growing demand for treatment and there is an increasing number of drug-induced illnesses which have to be treated. And, for the altruistic, possibly because holistic treatment increases the carer's contact with the patient, an interaction which modern high-tech developments seem to restrict.

Homoeopathy is the most widely used and easily available of the alternative systems of medicine. Incorporated in the NHS since 1948, it provides an excellent form of treatment for primary health-care. Many of the medicines used are appropriate for self-prescription in cases of minor, limited conditions; however, when prescribed by skilled practitioners they can also be used for chronic conditions – and may often be far more beneficial than the long-term treatments offered by orthodox medicine (the risks of side effects are extremely rare and homoeopathic medicines are definitely non-addictive).

It is for these reasons that many parents turn to homoeopathy when their children are taken ill. It is not a rejection of the conventional treatment offered by the doctor; it is the realisation that although orthodox medicine and modern life-saving technology have a place in our health-care management, these can be used as a last resort, when other, more gentle methods have failed.

It is encouraging that a greater choice of over-the-counter natural medicines is becoming available, and it is because of this that a good self-help book like *Homoeopathy for Babies and Children* becomes invaluable, if not essential. But a word of caution: self-prescription can only go so far, and without the training necessary to prescribe in the way appropriate to the therapy, the treatment is not holistic – the skill and expertise of the practitioner should not be forgotten.

When Beth MacEoin asked if I would like to write the foreword to *Homoeopathy for Babies and Children*, it raised the question, who were going to be the main readers? Parents! Parents with babies and young children. So I took the manuscript to a selection of parents for their views, some having a basic understanding of homoeopathy, others with little or none.

The response from all was exactly the same as my own: a well written, concise explanation of homoeopathy with easy-to-follow instruction charts and good, clear warnings and cautions. Beth leads the reader gently into building up the remedy 'picture', suggesting dosage instructions and giving information on what to expect after administering the remedy.

One of my 'guinea pig' parents, familiar with *Kent's Repertory* and a variety of homoeopathic self-help books, said that when one of her children became ill or had an accident, it would take her ages to find the indicated remedy. However, following Beth's tables had made it easier and quicker, whilst also explaining that you only need to look up the symptoms ('repertorise') of the differences, not the normal condition, of the child – something which she felt had never been explained properly in other books.

All in all, the assistance of the parents in 'road testing' the directions of the book proved to me that it worked in the way the author had hoped. *Homoeopathy for Babies and Children* is not aimed at turning the reader into an experienced and skilled homoeopath, but it is successfully directed at giving parents a clear understanding of the principles of homoeopathic prescribing for self-help and accident situations; that Beth, in addition, gives clear indications of when to consult the professional is very reassuring.

This is an informative, educational self-help guide that has the additional bonus of being an enjoyable read.

Sato Liu
The Natural Medicines Society
May 1994

ACKNOWLEDGEMENTS

Thanks are due to a number of people who have been immensely helpful while this book was being written. As always, my agent Teresa Chris has been a tremendous source of encouragement and moral support throughout. I am also extremely grateful to the editorial staff at Headway for their advice, patience and guidance during the production of the manuscript. Homoeopathic practitioners who must also be thanked for their suggestions and constructive advice on improvements on the text include Steven Gordon, April Jackson and Mirando Castro. I am also indebted to Sato Liu for her exceptional energy, sense of humour and sound common sense when presented with the manuscript at various stages for her comments.

My deepest thanks, as always, go to my husband Denis for being an exceptionally patient, good-humoured, and lovable companion while this book was in progress. Without his help and support, I am fully confident it would never have seen the light of day. Finally, thanks also to my mother Nancy for having carried out the demanding task of bringing me up with the most important quality a parent needs: an essential sense of fun.

Beth MacEoin

INTRODUCTION

The positive aspects of homoeopathic treatment for children

Homoeopathy provides an excellent system of health care for children: not only is it one of the most effective forms of holistic medicine available, but, used competently, it can restore a sick child to health in a swift, effective and untraumatic way, with the minimum risk of side effects.

Because children tend to have dramatic recuperative qualities, favourable responses to homoeopathic remedies are equivalently crisp and clear, which makes successful prescribing for children especially rewarding. Very young children's symptoms are also presented with more candour and clarity than those of an adult, partly because they are unaware of social conventions, but also because their symptoms have usually escaped the masking or suppressive effect of repeated courses of conventional drugs to which adults are so often subjected.

It is quite surprising to many people that age is no barrier to homoeopathic treatment: babies of a few weeks old can be treated as appropriately as the elderly. Most homoeopaths will say that there are few barriers to homoeopathy in treating illness but that there are certain individuals who respond more vigorously to treatment than others. Since well-established illness in a person who has been given long-term drug therapy can result in a favourable response being slow to come and more difficult to promote, we can see that a young child who has recently fallen ill within the context of good health is likely to be easier to treat.

Homoeopathic treatment has a particular application which makes it very relevant to treating children: this is the appropriateness of homoeopathy in dealing with childhood illnesses such as chicken-pox, whooping cough and measles. Since these illnesses are viral rather than bacterial in nature, there is little available from conventional medicine to help apart from painkillers and soothing lotions. Because homoeopathic medicines are understood to act by stimulating and assisting the body's own self-healing mechanism, it is irrelevant whether the illness is bacterial or viral. Once the appropriate homoeopathic medicine has acted, the body gets on with the job of dealing with the infection efficiently and with the minimum amount of complications, regardless of the nature of the disease-causing agent.

Homoeopathy is also very popular with parents who are worried about the potential side effects of routine or excessive use of conventional drugs, such as antibiotics, in young children. Where a condition has become chronic (subject to repeated flare-ups over an extended period of time, such as frequent ear infections or constant sore throats), homoeopathy has a great deal to offer in providing long-term treatment to strengthen the resilience and constitution of a young child. When this treatment is successful, parents are often delighted to find that their child throws off infections more quickly and decisively and falls ill less frequently. Most important of all, when homoeopathic treatment is effective on this profound level, parents often comment on their child exhibiting a greater sense of vitality and general well-being.

Homoeopathic medicine can also be immensely valuable in helping a child overcome acute (limited time-span) problems such as those listed in this book. The pain and distress of sore throats, vomiting, earache and teething can be eased swiftly and with the minimum of fuss once the most appropriate homoeopathic remedy has been selected and administered. It is an added bonus that there is rarely a struggle in administering homoeopathic remedies to children, since they usually love the taste of the lactose (milk sugar) base. As a beginner, it takes time, practice and a bit of confidence to prescribe effectively for straightforward children's problems, but you will find that the information given in this book will give you the basics with which to begin.

The information in this book is advisory in nature and should not be regarded as a replacement for the services of a health professional. If in doubt, consult your GP or homoeopathic practitioner. Neither the publishers nor the author accept responsibility for the consequences of self-treatment.

CHAPTER 1

THE BASICS OF HOMOEOPATHY

What is homoeopathic medicine?

Homoeopathy is a system of medicine which has existed for almost 200 years. It is practised worldwide by both conventional doctors and professional homoeopaths. In expert hands, it provides a way of restoring the sick person to good health in a gentle, thorough, balanced and effective manner.

The concept of similars

The word 'homoeopathy' comes from a Greek source, and means something like 'similar suffering'. In other words, a substance which in material doses causes disease in a healthy person can be used to therapeutic advantage in a sick person, provided his symptoms resemble those known to be produced by that substance. The concept of using similars was an idea which had existed from the time of the ancient Greek physician Hippocrates, but Samuel Hahnemann, an eighteenth-century physician and the originator of homoeopathy as a modern medical theory, took the basic concept much further by developing into it into a full medical system with a coherent philosophical basis. In doing so, he put forward an extremely controversial theory of health and disease which ran completely against the grain of the current medical thinking of his own day, and which continues to contradict orthodox concepts in the late twentieth century.

Instead of prescribing a medicine designed to control the symptoms of illness by counteracting them, Hahnemann recommended the use of medicines which worked by assisting and stimulating the body's own efforts to come to terms with disease. Disease itself he saw as merely the body's often fruitless attempt to react to external or internal stresses such as bacteria, viruses and toxins. By approaching the problem of illness from this perspective, Hahnemann developed a theory of healing which was more concerned with stimulating the body to work more effectively, than weakening it through violent measures such as bloodletting or purging (both of which were very fashionable in orthodox medical circles of his day).

Provings of remedies

In order to find out what effects a medicinal substance would have on a healthy individual, Hahnemann carried out a series of controlled experiments on himself and other volunteers. These experiments were called 'provings', and they involved taking small amounts of a substance repeatedly and recording the effects in minute detail. The people selected had to be in good health at the time of the experiment, and ready to observe and record very precisely any changes in their physical or emotional health for as long as it continued. Today, many hundreds of homoeopathic medicines are in use which have been proved in just this manner, and the process continues as new medicines are introduced. The accumulated information on each 'proved' medicine is used to produce profiles or pictures of each medicinal substance. These are used as reference material for selecting medicines for patients.

The single dose

Homoeopathic medicines are commonly given as single remedies in single doses because the original provings were carried out using simple substances rather than compounds. The reactions of the patient are noted, and the decision is made by the practitioner whether to wait, repeat, move to a lower or higher potency, or change the remedy altogether.

One of the strongest arguments which supports the administration of a single remedy is that it is very difficult to assess how effective a particular remedy has been if it is closely followed by, or even mixed with, another. Because of the tradition of proving single substances rather than compounds or mixtures, the information on therapeutic effects is also not available for multiple compounds, so the effects of the interaction between these substances is something we cannot be reliably aware of.

The minimum dose

As well as the concept of treating by similar agents, Hahnemann also developed the idea that the dose of the medicine given should be the smallest amount possible to stimulate a cure without side effects. This preoccupation can be traced back to the appalling effects from drugs that he witnessed during his career as an orthodox physician. He was, therefore, motivated to experiment using increasingly smaller doses of similar medicinal substances, until he came to a point of dilution where orthodox medical science parted company with him. Although no molecules of the original substance could be detected at this level of dilution, Hahnemann discovered that such highly dilute medicines had a profound effect in stimulating the self-healing properties of the body, provided they were subjected to an additional process of 'succussion' or vigorous shaking at each stage of dilution.

As long as the essential similarity between the medicine and the patient's symptoms was established, Hahnemann found that the more dilute and further away from a material dose a homoeopathic remedy became, the stronger and more potent the medicinal effect on the patient proved to be – always provided it had gone through succussion.

Therefore, in order for a substance to be considered to be homoeopathically active, three factors must be present:

- Serial dilution.
- Succussion.
- As close a match as possible between the symptoms of the sick person and information available regarding the action of the medicinal substance on the human system.

Homoeopathy treats people, not diseases

The concept of treating each patient as an individual who responds to illness in their own way is central to homoeopathic practice. Any changes or disturbances which have appeared on physical, emotional and mental levels since illness began must be paid attention to: it is an analysis of this vital information which will lead the practitioner to select the most appropriate homoeopathic medicine.

Although a basic diagnostic name can be given to a group of common symptoms, no two children or adults will suffer illness in quite the same way. In other words, even though they experience the same basic disease, their individual symptoms may be affected quite differently by common factors. If we take the simplest example of two children suffering from influenza, both will have general symptoms of feverishness, aching, lack of energy, sore throats, nasal discharge and coughs. However, this general information will not help the homoeopath in searching for the appropriate homoeopathic prescription, since it conveys nothing about the way each individual child is dealing with his or her illness.

In order to discover this, it is necessary to probe more deeply into the individualising characteristics of each child's symptoms, in order to see a sharper picture emerging. Once we begin to observe more closely, we may discover that one child fell ill very rapidly within a matter of hours and experienced a very quick rise in temperature. Since falling ill, all he wanted was to be left alone in a darkened room to try to relieve the severe headache that came on with the fever. Any stimulation from well-meaning relatives or friends would make him feel worse. Although terribly drowsy, he couldn't get to sleep because of pain in his head and his severe sore throat. Trying to drink would make the discomfort in his throat worse, and even though his mouth was very dry, he was not thirsty. His skin was bright red and dry, and so hot that it radiated heat that could be felt by anyone near to him.

The second child began to feel ill by complaining of a sore

throat that got progressively worse as the day went on. Her symptoms were much worse during the night, when she became unusually anxious, restless and fretful. Normally a very placid child who slept well, she could only be comforted by having someone with her all through the night. Once left alone, she became very distressed and anxious. Although she complained of burning in her throat, having regular sips of warm drinks was very soothing to her. She also complained of being terribly chilly and felt much better being kept very warm. Although feverish during the night, she looked pale and tired rather than flushed.

In these two elementary examples we can see straight away how each child is expressing symptoms in his or her own individual way. It would be of little help to give the same homoeopathic remedy to both of them, since their specific symptoms are quite different (even though they share general features of the illness). Unless a close match exists between the symptoms of a homoeopathic remedy and the symptoms of the sick person, no amount of an inappropriately chosen medicine will be of any help at all in stimulating self-healing. In this case, the first child would be given Belladonna, and the second Arsenicum album. This is because it is the sick child who is being prescribed for, not the abstract disease category of influenza.

Homoeopathy and conventional medicine

In order to understand fully the marked contrast between the homoeopathic and orthodox medical view of health and disease, we need to look at the context within which Samuel Hahnemann developed his ideas.

The early days of homoeopathy

Samuel Hahnemann was born in 1755 in Meissen, Germany and qualified as a doctor in 1779. The more he witnessed of the medical procedures that were fashionable at that time, such as leeching, cupping, purging through vast quantities of laxatives, and the use of highly toxic substances such as Mercury to treat venereal disease, the more convinced he became that he was doing more harm than good by practising as an orthodox physician.

As a result, in 1796 Hahnemann decided to stop practising as a physician and put his efforts into translating foreign medical texts. He also began to conduct experiments of his own into gentler and less barbaric ways of treating patients.

While translating Cullen's *Materia Medica*, he was intrigued and perplexed by the author's explanation for the effectiveness of Cinchona (Peruvian bark) as a medicinal substance in treating the symptoms of malaria. The explanation given by Cullen, that it was the astringent properties of Cinchona which rendered it medicinally effective, did not satisfy Hahnemann, who decided that he would conduct some experiments of his own in order to see if another explanation presented itself. The experiment which followed involved Hahnemann's taking repeated doses of Cinchona himself, and observing the effects. He found that while he continued to take doses of Cinchona, he began to develop symptoms of malaria which went away once he stopped taking the medicine. As a direct result of this insight, he began the long and tortuous path of developing the philosophy and practice of homoeopathy: the treatment of sick individuals with similar substances rather than opposites. Hahnemann emphatically believed that the latter would merely suppress the symptoms of illness by temporarily promoting an opposite action rather than supporting the body to heal itself. He continued to develop and refine his ideas and their practical application until his death in Paris in 1843.

After working further along these lines with a broader range of medicinal substances, Hahnemann began to turn his attention to the problem of how to lessen any adverse effects that administration of the medicines caused. He began by using more and more dilute forms of medicine in an effort to produce the gentlest and most humane form of treatment. Then came a point where he made a quantum leap in his thinking by adding the systematic repetition of vigorous shaking or 'succussion' at each stage of dilution. He found that these twin procedures had to be carried out in order for a medicine to be suitable for homoeopathic use. This process came to be called 'potentization'.

The more he observed the effects of these potentized medicinal substances, the more he discovered that his observations ran counter to anything that could be explained by the scientific theories of his day. From the reactions he observed in his patients, the more dilute and succussed a medicine became (even to the point where there was no remaining molecule of the original substance present), the more powerful the effect appeared to be on the sick person, provided the 'similarity' of the patient's symptom picture as a whole matched that of the prescribed remedy.

Homoeopathy and vital energy

While Hahnemann developed and refined his ideas, he concluded that there must be some basic intelligence which presided over the harmonious functioning of the human body in a balanced state of health. When this 'vital force' or basic intelligence came in contact with a stressful stimulus which it could not resist, symptoms of illness or disease would start to appear in the individual. These symptoms would be a sign of the body's own dynamic, but ineffective, attempt to promote self-healing, thus giving clues as to the nature of the imbalance, and also providing vital information for the selection of the appropriate homoeopathic remedy.

If we take this approach, symptoms of illness acquire a more benign role from a homoeopathic standpoint than a conventional medical perspective.

Health and disease and orthodox medicine

Modern medicine views the human body as constantly under siege from hostile invaders such as bacteria and viruses, and, as a result, many drug companies work along the lines of searching for the 'magic bullet' which will fight and eliminate the offending microbe. In contrast to homoeopathy, which stimulates and strengthens the body's own self-healing capacity to overcome infection, conventional medicine works by identifying the individual organism through investigations and tests, in order to eliminate it by giving the appropriate drug.

Conventional drugs are also very different in preparation

and prescription when compared with the homoeopathic selection of medicines. Because homoeopathic remedies work by stimulating the body's self-defence mechanism, they enable it to fight disease more effectively. Orthodox or 'allopathic' drugs, however, work in quite a different way, since they are chosen on the basis of their counteracting disease symptoms by producing an opposite effect. Examples with which we are familiar include the use of antacids to counter over-acidity in the stomach, laxatives for constipation, antibiotics to eliminate bacteria, and anti-inflammatories to reduce inflammation. Because drugs such as these work by counteracting symptoms, they need to be taken on a long-term basis in order to keep the symptoms under control.

The homoeopathic approach differs by concentrating on aiding the body to work more efficiently so that it can come to terms with, and overcome, symptoms itself. Homoeopaths see the human body as having an in-built self-healing capacity which, when working efficiently and harmoniously, fights off infection very effectively. However, if this system is put under excessive strain for too long, symptoms begin to emerge which will not clear up of their own accord. By giving an appropriately-chosen homoeopathic remedy it is possible to stimulate the body's self-healing capacity once again so that it is able to resolve the situation effectively and decisively. As a result, the long-term aim of successful homoeopathic treatment is to get the body in a sufficient degree of balance so that further intervention is unnecessary unless, or until, the body is further overwhelmed by stress.

Limitations of conventional medicine

One of the main drawbacks of conventional treatment is the emphasis given to common disease symptoms in the search for the appropriate drug therapy. As a result, it is easy to lose sight of the individual person in pursuit of diagnosis. This often leads to the ill person feeling they are little more than an animated disease label: a feeling which is unfortunately unwittingly reinforced by the battery of investigative procedures to which they may be exposed.

Because conventional medicine regards good health as the absence of disease, rather than the positive acquisition of a healthy and well-balanced body, we have been educated to expect a pill to deal with each minor problem that may surface with regard to our health. This is often the result of many doctors losing sight of the human body as an integrated system with a defence mechanism of its own, which, when healthy, can fight off illness very effectively. Consequently, we have lost touch with the basic knowledge we can use to aid ourselves or our children through short-term infections like the common cold. Sensible supportive measures such as increasing fluid intake, keeping food light and digestible, resting and keeping in as even a temperature as possible, especially while feverish, are all common-sense measures which help the body fight infection. Unfortunately, many of us will take pills to mask unpleasant symptoms temporarily in order to keep going, only to find that we take longer to recover with a higher risk of developing complications. This is the legacy of the magic bullet, which encourages us to ignore or suppress the important message our body is sending us: that we may need to take it easy for a few days.

When homoeopathy is used effectively, it supports adults

and children through the stages of illness quickly and with the minimum risk of complications. If we take the common cold as an example, judicious homoeopathic prescribing is unlikely to stop the illness in its tracks, but it can speed up the progress of cure and make the risk of extended chest or sinus problems less likely. Because homoeopathy works by assisting the body in its attempt to resolve disease, any further measures that support this fight will be of value. This is why you will find listed in each chapter of this book a large measure of general advice, as well as tables which give you the basic information you need regarding relevant homoeopathic remedies for each condition.

CHAPTER 2

HOMOEOPATHY IN ACTION

Conditions which are appropriate for home prescribing

In the following chapters you will find a range of children's conditions listed which can respond effectively and decisively to self-help measures and homoeopathic prescribing. These include short-term illnesses such as stomach upsets, sore throats, colds, and situations requiring homoeopathic first-aid, such as cuts and bruises. Within this context, results obtained can be exciting, rapid and reassuringly gentle.

Children's conditions that do not lend themselves to home prescribing are listed in Chapter 7, Chronic and Long-term Problems in Children. You will find within this section a basic explanation highlighting why chronic conditions, such as eczema, asthma or recurrent ear infections, should be taken to a homoeopathic practitioner rather than attempting to treat such problems yourself. Homoeopathy has a great deal to offer children in this situation, especially where parents are concerned about possible side effects of long-term conventional medication and wish to explore more holistic alternatives. However, it must be stressed that managing a long-term or well-established disorder in a child requires the experience, objectivity and theoretical knowledge of a homoeopathic practitioner to ensure the most positive outcome possible.

Care should also be taken with any of the conditions listed in this book as suitable for home prescribing, if they show signs of more serious complications, or if you suspect your child is getting worse. You will find suggestions at the end of each section which indicate that your child might require professional help. Within this context, such help should come from your General Practitioner (GP), or, in very severe emergencies where time is short, the emergency department of your nearest hospital. In less urgent situations, existing patients of a professional or doctor homoeopath should notify their practitioner of the situation. If you do not have immediate access to a homoeopathic practitioner, you can contact your GP initially, and after the immediate emergency has been dealt with, consider finding a homoeopathic practitioner to investigate the problem more deeply.

Although your child may not have the exact symptoms listed under the suggestions which alert you to the need for professional help, always follow your instinct if you suspect your child is becoming gravely ill. This may be based on your observation of an altered feeding pattern or uncharacteristic crying in a baby, severe and rapidly advancing lethargy or marked change in behaviour in an older child. Remember that, although they are very resilient, young babies and children can become very ill with alarming rapidity, and you should always seek expert advice promptly if you suspect this may be the case.

Using this book

Selecting the right remedy

In order to obtain the most satisfactory results when using this book, you need to do the following:

• Write down any symptoms you have noticed since the onset of illness. With babies or small children who cannot communicate verbally, you will need to use your senses as much as possible to put together relevant information. Listen to any changes in your child's breathing or cry, feel any changes in the texture of your child's skin, look at your child's complexion regarding uncharacteristic paleness or flushing, and smell any changes in odour with regard to your child's breath, urine, sweat or stools. Most of all, be alert to any changes in your child's behaviour regarding feeding, sleeping, or uncharacteristic changes of mood.

• Remember you are only interested in changes from the normal, healthy state of your child. In other words, if your toddler is normally on the pale and chilly side when healthy, but since falling ill has been persistently red-faced and sensitive to heat, this would be a valid symptom because it signifies a change from the normal state of your child.

• Once you have a complete list of symptoms you regard as important, highlight any that you regard as being peculiar. For example, nausea that is relieved by eating, chilliness with aversion to heat, or fever without thirst. These are very valuable symptoms that may be the deciding factor in helping you choose the most appropriate remedy.

• Identify a characteristic theme or general feature running through your child's symptoms. For instance, burning or redness could be a characteristic of discharges, sore throats, or general pains, or dryness could be a common feature of skin texture, sensations in mouth or throat, and bowel movements. When you have a common theme like this running through the major symptoms, it becomes easier to identify the most appropriate remedy. This is because you will have less of a sense of prescribing for a 'rag bag' of unrelated symptoms, and more of a sense of compiling a symptom picture which hangs together.

• Consider if there has been a precipitating factor before the onset of illness, such as exposure to cold winds, a severe fright or shock, or several nights of disturbed sleep.

• Take note of anything that makes your child feel generally better or worse. This can apply to anything which relieves or aggravates individual symptoms, or which has a general effect on improving or aggravating your child.

• Always pay attention to any emotional changes which have occurred before or since illness set in. Anxiety in a placid child, weepiness in a cheerful and resilient child, or restlessness and anxiety in a usually relaxed child, are always symptoms of great value.

• By now you should have a fairly comprehensive list of symptoms which you can divide under headings of causitive factors, general symptoms and modalities (things which generally make your child worse or better).

• Remember that the general symptom heading can have a very wide scope, referring to any changes on both physical and emotional levels.

• You are now ready to turn to the appropriate table in the relevant section of this book. Look down the left-hand column entitled *Type* to identify which category fits most closely with the group of symptoms you have on paper. If you have a causitive factor to work with at this stage, it will be of great help to you. This column also provides you with information regarding the stage of your child's illness, for instance, whether you are looking for symptoms relating to early onset of illness, or a more established stage.

• When you have settled on the category that seems most appropriate, check the information given under the next column entitled *General Indications* to see if these correspond with those of your child. It is unlikely that you will find a perfect match between the two, so don't worry if you can't find all the symptoms you have noted under this heading. What you must assess is whether the essential elements of the general indications cover the most characteristic and prominent symptoms of your child. For instance, you would not consider Aconite unless your child was in the early stage of a rapidly developing fever, with marked restlessness, flushed face, strong anxiety leading to panic, with most symptoms developing or getting worse as the night goes on. If your child had a slowly developing fever which took days to emerge, looked pale, with-drawn and quiet, and just wanted to be left as still as possible, Aconite would be quite unsuitable and you would need to look elsewhere for the appropriate remedy.

• Be creative in how you use the remedy tables. For example, if your child has a cold with a sore throat and cough, you can combine information from each of these separate tables in order to broaden your choice, and expand the amount of information available to you.

• If you are unsure which symptoms represent essen-tial features of a homoeopathic remedy, turn to the section at the back of the book entitled **Keynotes**. This will give you a quick tour of the essential characteristics running through each remedy.

• When you are satisfied that the match between your child's symptoms and the homoeopathic remedy you are considering are close enough, look at the *Worse from* and *Better for* columns. If you feel that these also apply to your child since illness began, then you can be quite confident that you have selected the most appro-priate remedy.

• Bear in mind that you are looking for the informa-tion that characterises what is individual in the symp-toms of your child. Always try to find out what is unique to your child's stomach upset or influenza. Common symptoms such as vomiting, diarrhoea, sore throat or cough will not help you choose between different remedies. You must always try to establish how these broad symptoms affect your child as an individual in the way they experience pain, the colour and texture of their discharges, and how these specific symptoms affect their systems as a whole.

• After using the tables for a while, you will notice that some medicines appear in more than one section. For instance, Arsenicum album appears in the tables for coughs, influenza and food poisoning, while Pulsatilla appears in tables for earache, chicken-pox and German measles. As you use these tables and refer to the **Keynotes** at the back of the book, you will begin to see that these are multi-faceted medicines that cover a wide range of complaints in their own individual way. Over time, as you become more familiar with their use, you will begin to appreciate how each remedy has its own individual characteristics, in the same way that your child has his or her own unique personality.

Giving homoeopathic medicines to children

• One of the most positive aspects of homoeopathic treatment with regard to children, is that they love the taste of the remedies. As a result, there is rarely a struggle in giving a child the appropriate medicine: in fact, they usually can't wait for the next dose! Although homoeopathic medicines are usually given in tablet form, they can also be administered as pilules, granules, liquids or powders, or applied to the skin in creams, diluted tinctures or ointments.

• When you have selected the appropriate remedy for your child, tip out a single dose (one tablet) on a clean spoon.

• You do not need to halve the dose for a child. It is

the potency and frequency of repetition of the selected remedy that determines the strength and length of its action, rather than the size of the dose. In other words, if you give one, two or ten tablets at the same time it still counts as a single dose of the remedy. However, if you gave a single tablet to your child every ten minutes over the course of an hour, this would count as six doses, since the remedy is being given repeatedly.

• Get your child to suck the remedy as they would a sweet, or if they get bored, they can chew it. Small children or babies can be given their remedy in granule or powder form, or you can make your own finely ground powder by crushing one tablet between two clean spoons. Then take a pinch of the remedy and place it under the tongue to be dissolved, or rub it on your child's gums.

• Ensure that your child has as clean a mouth as possible when taking their remedy. Bear in mind that a clean mouth does not involve brushing your child's teeth before giving their medicine, but refers more to ensuring that they have not eaten or drunk anything that has a strong flavour, such as mint, too close to taking their remedy. As a basic guide, allow half an hour either side of eating or drinking.

• Substances that are thought to interfere with the medicinal action of homoeopathic remedies include peppermint, tea, coffee, or strong-smelling menthol or camphor rubs. Aromatic oils such as Olbas Oil should also be avoided when using remedies. If you are a beginner in home-prescribing, it is a good idea to ensure your child steers clear of any of these while taking their remedy. This avoids an element of potential confusion if it looks like the selected remedy is not working.

• Store your remedies away from strong light, strong smells and extreme heat and cold. A fairly cool, dark place is most suitable (not in the fridge). If you keep homoeopathic medicines under these conditions they will remain medicinally active, since they have a long shelf-life if stored well.

• If you have an accident and spill some tablets out of the bottle, do not put them back in; throw them away since they may have been damaged.

One dose or two? Deciding how often to repeat your child's remedy

• After you have given your child the first dose of an indicated remedy (a single dose being one tablet), wait for half an hour. If you observe no change, repeat the remedy. You can repeat the same remedy for up to three doses at intervals of half an hour.

• If you notice any signs of improvement after the first, second or third dose, stop giving the remedy. This improvement is a sign that your child's body is now doing the job of resolving the illness by itself, and continuing to give the remedy at this stage is unnecessary. If your child relapses, and the same symptoms recur, you will need to resume giving the remedy in the same way as before. Once again, as soon as you see an improvement, stop giving the remedy.

- The instructions outlined above are recommendations for repetition of the appropriate remedy in a condition of sudden and recent onset, as in a case of stomach upset or earache. However, if your child's symptoms have been slowly developing over a few days, and appear to be less vigorous and more stubborn, she is likely to respond more favourably to repetition of the appropriate remedy three times daily over the course of two or three days. As before, do not give the remedy routinely, but stop as soon as you see an initial or continued improvement.

- If there is no improvement after waiting the suggested time, take a fresh look at the table you have been using and see if another remedy is more suitable. If one remedy hasn't worked, there is no problem of incompatibility of medicines in moving on to another which may be more effective. Because the remedies are working at a sub-molecular level, there is no risk of any chemical residue being left in your child's system which might spark off a toxic reaction.

- If your child's condition is fairly mild and of recent onset, you can begin by giving the selected remedy in a 6c (see the discussion on potencies on page 140) potency. If you see some improvement after giving the remedy as instructed, but feel that you have to keep on giving it to maintain an improvement, move on to the same remedy in a 12c. You can begin with a 12c or 30c potency (both are available from homoeopathic pharmacies) if your child's condition has been of longer duration or if the symptoms are more intense.

- Bear in mind that the self-help application of

homoeopathic remedies as outlined within the context of this book is for short-term use only. If you feel that you need to give them on a daily basis to your child to achieve and maintain the desired effect, you should seek more long-term 'constitutional', treatment from a homoeopathic practitioner. For further details regarding why this is necessary see Chapter 7: Chronic and Long-Term Problems in Children.

• Most important of all, if you feel your child is not responding to homoeopathic prescribing or general self-help measures, or if you suspect that he seems seriously ill, **always get medical advice promptly.**

CHAPTER 3

ACCIDENTS AND INJURIES

With the best will in the world, it is impossible to ensure that children do not have the occasional accident. Even if the best and most responsible precautions have been taken, children are experts in finding ways around these measures! As a result, falls, cuts and bruises can be a regular feature in a small child's life.

Bearing this in mind, homoeopathic prescribing and basic first-aid treatment used within this context can play a very positive role in minimising shock, speeding up the healing process and guarding against infection. It is also very helpful for a parent to feel there is something positive they can do to help their child beyond using basic first-aid measures such as bandaging or using cream on a wound.

In a situation where a minor accident has occurred, an appropriately chosen homoeopathic medicine acts as a catalyst, speeding up the processes which would naturally happen in the body, given enough time. The beneficial effect of homoeopathic treatment in falls and injuries can also be wide-reaching as in the use of Arnica, which not only deals with the initial shock sustained, but also limits bruising by encouraging re-absorption of blood, and minimising pain. Symphytum promotes the knitting of fractured bones and also reduces pain, while Calendula acts as a natural antiseptic, slows down bleeding and assists the healing of skin.

How to select the appropriate homoeopathic medicine

If your child has suffered a sprain, this is how you select the appropriate homoeopathic remedy:

• Turn to the table entitled **Sprains and Strains**, and look down the left-hand column in order to identify which category is most appropriate with regard to your child's symptoms. If, for example, your child feels much more comfortable for keeping the injured area still, it is likely that the column entitled '*Sprains and Strains* which are worse for the slightest movement' will be the most suitable.

• Check with the *General Indications* in the next column that the symptoms described also fit with those experienced by your child. If the joint looks inflamed and red and reacts badly to the slightest movement, but feels better for firm pressure, you are moving along the right lines. You can compare this information with other descriptions within General Indications in order to confirm your choice, or consider other possible remedies.

• Finally, check the *Worse from* and *Better for* columns in order to confirm that these also fit. Do bear in mind that these do not just apply to what makes your child's injury feel better or worse, but also what makes your child generally feel better or worse. If you find that the information in the **Keynotes** at the back of the book confirms your choice, (e.g. Bryonia) it will be the most appropriate remedy to try first.

- You will find that homoeopathic prescribing for accidents and injuries is different to other sections included within this book. This is because initial prescribing is much more routine for many conditions included in this chapter. For example, you will notice very quickly that Arnica is always recommended as the first remedy to take internally if there has been shock, trauma, bleeding or bruising following an injury. In many cases, you may need to select another remedy later which needs more careful differentiation if Arnica has helped a great deal in the initial stages, but improvement has stopped or symptoms have changed. Good examples would include fractures, strains or pain following dental work, all of which may require other remedies to resolve the situation.

For information on how to administer the selected remedy, see the section entitled *Giving homoeopathic medicines to children* in Chapter 2; exactly the same principles apply.

Remember that in first-aid situations you can give the appropriate remedy internally, while you are also applying the same, or another remedy, to the skin in the form of diluted tincture, cream, ointment or lotion. For example, if your child has fallen and grazed herself, it is fine to give Arnica internally while the grazes are bathed and cleaned with diluted Calendula tincture. You can follow this with applying Calendula ointment directly to the graze, or put it on a clean dressing and apply this to the injured area. Always remember that Arnica cream should **never** be applied to bruises where the skin has been broken; only those where the skin is intact. In the former situation, Calendula or a combination of Hypericum and Calendula is the most appropriate choice of ointment or cream.

Cuts and bruises

TYPE	GENERAL INDICATIONS	WORSE FROM	BETTER FOR	REMEDY NAME
Simple cuts and bruises	Straightforward cuts, bruises and abrasions which show no signs of sepsis. Apply the remedy to the skin in diluted tincture, lotion, cream or ointment.	Chill	Being still	Calendula
Deep cuts and incised wounds with nerve involvement	Especially indicated where areas rich in nerve supply have been crushed or damaged. These include fingers, toes, and soles of feet. Shooting pains with hypersensitivity to touch.	Movement. Touch	Keeping still	Hypericum
Incised wounds with hyper-sensitivity to pain	Useful in treating shock and pain of clean cuts with stinging, lacerated sensations. Often needed after injury from sharp instruments.	Movement. Pressure	Heat. Resting	Staphy-sagria
Early stage of simple bruising with restlessness	General state of emotional and physical shock following accident or injury. Soreness and aching with bruising. Arnica cream or ointment can also be applied to the skin **provided there is no sign of a cut or graze.**	Touch. Exertion	Resting	Arnica

27

TYPE	GENERAL INDICATIONS	WORSE FROM	BETTER FOR	REMEDY NAME
Bruises and black eyes that are relieved by cold compresses	Indicated after Arnica has ceased to ease pain and discomfort of bruised tissue. Pains feel tearing, stabbing or pulling and are accompanied by tense, hard swelling of the skin.	Heat. Moving	Cold bathing. Cool air. Resting	Ledum
Bruising that follows injury to eyeball or eye socket	Strongly indicated if eye has been injured by a blunt object. Very helpful in situations where Arnica has initially dealt with swelling around the eye, but pain remains.	Touch		Symphytum
Bruises where bones are covered by a thin layer of skin: elbows and shins.	Sore, lame and bruised pains. Very strongly indicated for bruises and damage involving the periosteum (the membranous sheath that covers bones).	Sitting. Going up or down stairs. Lying on injured area	Warmth. Rubbing	Ruta
Deep bruising	Indicated after a blow that causes bruising of deep tissue, e.g. after a bad fall or blow to the chest.	Touch. Hot bathing	Cold compresses	Bellis perennis

General advice

The following first-aid measures will be necessary in addition to homoeopathic prescribing:

- In any injury where the skin has been broken, gently bathe the wound making sure you remove any visible dirt. Before applying a sterile dressing, examine the wound carefully to check that no embedded dirt has been left in the skin.
- If you are bathing a cut or graze, use diluted Calendula or a combination of Hypericum and Calendula tincture to clean the wound. Either will make an excellent antiseptic solution when diluted in cooled, boiled water. Make sure you do not apply the tincture 'neat' to grazed skin, because it will sting; dilute one part of tincture to ten parts of water. Calendula is extremely effective in speeding up healing of lacerated skin, helps to stop bleeding and acts as a natural antiseptic making the complication of infection less likely.
- After bathing the wound as described above, apply Calendula or Hypericum and Calendula cream or ointment to the wound. Use cream for simple cuts and ointment for rough or grazed skin.
- If the skin is intact and the area bruised and swollen, apply cold compresses to the injured part for twenty to thirty minutes in order to ease pain and reduce inflammation.
- If the skin is **not** broken, apply Arnica cream or ointment to the bruised area. This will act together with internal administration of the remedy to relieve pain and speed up the healing process.

When to seek medical advice
If any of the following occur, seek professional help:

- Bleeding which is profuse or accompanied by tingling, numbness or loss of strength.
- Deep cuts to face, chest or abdomen, or wide cuts which will not be held together by adhesive bandage.
- Dirt or other foreign bodies which cannot be removed from a wound by bathing.
- Signs of infection anywhere, especially on the palms of the hands or the undersides of the fingers.
- Repeated, easy bruising.
- If the area of bruising is extensive, or the result of a severe blow. This is especially important if an eye, or the surrounding tissue, is involved.

Puncture wounds

TYPE	GENERAL INDICATIONS	WORSE FROM	BETTER FOR	REMEDY NAME
Puncture wounds which feel much better for cold bathing	Pains are stinging, throbbing and pricking. Wound looks red and swollen but feels cold when touched. Pain and swelling greatly relieved by cold bathing. Unless symptoms suggest otherwise, this is the first remedy to consider in puncture wounds.	Warmth	Cold bathing	Ledum

TYPE	GENERAL INDICATIONS	WORSE FROM	BETTER FOR	REMEDY NAME
Puncture wounds with marked puffy, pink, swollen skin	Site of the wound looks very swollen: almost as though water were trapped beneath the skin. Very hot around the injury with stinging pains. The affected area feels much worse for exposure to heat in any form.	Heat. Touch	Cool air. Cold bathing	Apis
Shooting, sharp pains with puncture wounds	Affected area is hypersensitive to touch. Lacerating pains that radiate or shoot along the affected limb from the site of injury.	Touch. Jarring		Hypericum

General advice

The following first-aid advice will be helpful in addition to homoeopathic prescribing:

• Clean the wound as thoroughly as possible, ensuring that it bleeds for a while to aid the removal of foreign bodies or debris. If bleeding is severe, apply pressure to the appropriate point above the artery, but ensure that you avoid putting pressure on the wound itself, otherwise there is a danger of pushing any foreign bodies deeper into the wound.

• Soak the wounded area in warm water in order to bring blood to the area (if there has been very little bleeding), and also to encourage the elimination of foreign bodies or

germs. Use diluted Hypericum and Calendula tincture in
the water.

- Apply diluted Hypericum and Calendula tincture to the
wound in order to speed up healing and to ease pain, as
well as giving the appropriate homoeopathic remedy
internally.

When to seek medical advice
If any of the following occur, seek professional help:

- Signs of infection around a puncture wound.
- Deep puncture wounds, or those located anywhere apart
from the extremities (hands, feet, etc).
- Puncture wounds which affect the hands rather than the
fingers, or puncture wounds to a joint, especially if you see
any sign of infection.
- Get professional advice promptly if you suspect the onset
of tetanus. Symptoms include rigidity of the injured limb
and painful spasms of the muscles of the abdomen and spine.

Bleeding

TYPE	GENERAL INDICATIONS	WORSE FROM	BETTER FOR	REMEDY NAME
Bleeding associated with a fall or injury	General trauma and shock associated with an accident. This is the first remedy to consider in injury of any kind. Also an important remedy which promotes the re-absorption of blood where bruising has taken place.	Slight touch or contact	Lying down	Arnica

TYPE	GENERAL INDICATIONS	WORSE FROM	BETTER FOR	REMEDY NAME
Nose bleeds and small wounds that bleed excessively	Profuse nose bleeds that occur from over-vigorous blowing of the nose, or from a blow to the same area. Bleeding occurs very easily. Very anxious and in need of reassurance with bleeding.	Any exertion	Cold water. Open air. Reassurance	Phosphorus
Faintness and signs of shock with bleeding	State of near-collapse with bleeding. Skin feels cold, clammy and looks pale or greyish. Marked preference for cool air or being fanned. Nature of bleeding is oozing and steady.	Warmth	Cool air. Being fanned	Carbo veg
Nausea with bleeding and possible shortness of breath	Cold sweat accompanies bleeding, and a deathly nausea which feels much worse for the slightest movement. Nature of bleeding is bright red and gushing.	Warmth. Movement of any kind	Open air. Rest. Keeping as still as possible	Ipecac

General advice

The following first-aid advice will be helpful in addition to homoeopathic prescribing:

- Remember that a child's body contains a smaller amount of blood than an adult's, so that the consequences of major blood loss in a child are more serious than the same amount of bleeding in an adult. If bleeding is severe, get help quickly.

- Reassure your child as much as possible, especially if the sight of blood makes him feel sick and panicky.

- Avoid removing anything from a deep wound: if it is deeply-embedded it may be acting as a barrier against further blood loss. If it is removed, bleeding could become uncontrollable. If this should happen, seek medical help immediately.

- Put a clean pad over the wound and apply pressure to try to stop the bleeding. If something is embedded in the injured area, you will need to apply pressure around the wound to prevent pushing the object further in.

- Bandage the dressing in place firmly enough to control bleeding, but not so tight that it interferes with circulation to fingers or toes (if this is the case, they will turn blue).

- If bleeding comes through the bandage, keep it in place and put a fresh one on top. On no account remove the first one.

- If your child has a nose bleed, get her to lean well forward and make sure that she breathes through her mouth as you pinch the soft part of her nose. Get her to spit out any blood from her mouth to avoid the possibility of vomiting. If nose bleeds follow from an injury to the head, get professional advice.

When to seek medical advice
If any of the following occur, you must get professional help quickly:

- Signs of shock including any of the following:
  - Pallor (pale, grey or bluish-tinged skin).
  - Clammy, cold skin.

- Rapid or weak pulse.
- Yawning, panting or gasping for air.
- Confusion or unconsciousness.
- Marked thirst with any of the above.
- Breathing difficulties.
- If you suspect your child has sustained an injury causing internal bleeding.
- If injury has resulted in multiple wounds to one limb, or if you cannot stop blood flow from an injury.

Sprains and strains

TYPE	GENERAL INDICATIONS	WORSE FROM	BETTER FOR	REMEDY NAME
First stage with swelling and bruised pain	Inflammation, swelling and bruising. Pain much worse for movement. Useful for general shock associated with injury, or strain after over-exertion.	Touch. Moving	Keeping still	Arnica
Sprains and strains that feel better after continued movement	Pain follows initial movement, but once moving, feels much better. Injured area better for warmth, worse for cold. Restless with pain, especially at night. Often needed once initial stage of injury has passed.	At night. Exposure to cold and damp. Initial movement	Warmth in general. Warm bathing. Continued motion	Rhus tox

TYPE	GENERAL INDICATIONS	WORSE FROM	BETTER FOR	REMEDY NAME
Strains and sprains that are much worse for any movement	Hot, rosy-red swelling around site of injury. Stitching pains that are worse for heat. Where the symptoms agree, Bryonia follows well after Arnica has dealt with the initial situation.	Slight motion. Continued motion. Light touch. Warmth	Firm pressure. Keeping injured area as still as possible	Bryonia
Later stage of torn ligaments and tendons	Affinity for injured wrist and ankle joints. Pains are bruised and aching, and swelling may have originally been relieved by Arnica and Rhus tox. Pains worse from cold and lying on affected part.	Cold. Resting. Touch. Walking out of doors	Warmth. Moving about indoors	Ruta
Sprains that are relieved by cool bathing	Although injured area feels cool, pain is relieved by cold compresses and cool bathing. Pains associated with lots of stiffness: can only be moved after cold bathing. Extreme pain with injury.	Heat. Walking. At night	Cool bathing. Rest	Ledum

General advice

The following first-aid advice will be helpful in addition to homoeopathic prescribing:

- Keep the injured area as still as possible while you place an ice bag or cold pack over the painful part. Do not apply an ice-pack to skin where the surface has been broken.
- Put an elastic bandage over and above the injured area to immobilise the joint and assist in reducing swelling.
- Raise the injured limb to encourage drainage of body fluids and to reduce inflammation.
- Use warmth after cold compresses have ceased to be of use (usually necessary after the first twenty-four or forty-eight hours of cold packs). Warm compresses and bathing can feel soothing as well as encouraging elimination of excess fluid and helping to reduce inflammation.
- If injury to a joint is mild, gentle massage may feel soothing.
- Encourage your child to rest the injured area as much as possible since early, or over-use, of injured tendons and ligaments can cause further damage.

When to seek medical advice
If any of the following occur, seek professional advice:

- Blueness, coldness or numbness of the injured limb.
- Be especially careful with children who fall on an outstretched hand and injure their wrist. Fractures of the wrist bones often happen this way, and specialist

knowledge is needed to diagnose a fracture as opposed to a strain or sprain.

- Marked swelling or pain which does not respond to first-aid measures.
- If the joint cannot be straightened or if there are signs of looseness or distortion of the injured area.
- If your child cannot use a joint, or if it will not bear any weight twelve or twenty-four hours after the injury occurred.

Fractures

TYPE	GENERAL INDICATIONS	WORSE FROM	BETTER FOR	REMEDY NAME
As soon as the fracture has occurred	General symptoms of shock, trauma and local tenderness. Child may look dazed after injury and reject help and comfort as a reflex action in shock. Bruising and swelling around the damaged area.	Touch. Being approached	Resting	Arnica
Severe pain with fracture but little swelling	Violent aches and pains with generalised feelings of shock and weakness. Withdrawn with pain.	Pressure to injured area. Cold	Being disturbed	Eupatorium perfoliatum

TYPE	GENERAL INDICATIONS	WORSE FROM	BETTER FOR	REMEDY NAME
Fractures which have been set in place	Appropriate where initial pain and swelling have subsided, and the knitting of bone needs to be speeded up. Always make sure that bones have been set in correct alignment before giving this remedy.	Touch		Symphytum
Slow-knitting fractures, even after Symphytum has been given	Bones which are slow to knit with pain, numbness and stiffness of fractured limb.	Cold	Warmth. Rest	Calc phos

General advice

The following first-aid advice will be helpful in addition to homoeopathic prescribing:

- If you suspect your child has fractured a limb make sure that you keep the injured area as still as possible while you get professional help. Signs of fracture include:
  - Swelling
  - Pain on slight touch or movement
  - Distortion of the injured part
- Do not apply pressure or needlessly move any part of the body you suspect may be fractured. This can cause further injury and can result in shock.
- If the skin is unbroken, use cold packs to keep the swelling down.

When to seek professional advice
If any of the following occur, seek professional help:

- Any signs of shock. These include:
  - Faintness.
  - Clammy skin.
  - Pale or bluish tinge to the skin.
- Unconsciousness.
- Serious injuries to the neck, back, thigh or pelvis.
- Severe bruising or bleeding under the skin around the site of injury.
- **Whenever** you suspect a fracture has occurred, always get medical attention.

Burns

TYPE	GENERAL INDICATIONS	WORSE FROM	BETTER FOR	REMEDY NAME
First degree burns	Burns with redness, stinging, and burning. The remedy should be given internally, and can also be applied to the affected skin in **diluted** tincture or cream. Also consider Calendula or Combudoron (TM) diluted tincture, lotion or ointment.	Touch		Urtica urens

TYPE	GENERAL INDICATIONS	WORSE FROM	BETTER FOR	REMEDY NAME
Second degree burns	Blistering burns that are stinging and red.			Use Hypericum tincture diluted, and Urtica urens as an internal remedy. Once blisters have broken, change to diluted Calendula tincture.
Severe second degree burns	Large, acute blisters with rawness, burning, cutting and smarting. Pain and inflammation are violently acute.	Warmth. Movement	Cold	Cantharis
Severe second degree burns	Trembling with drawing, tearing pains. Indicated for effects of deep burns, or resolving old burns that are still causing pain	Draught	Even temperatures	Causticum

General advice

In addition to homoeopathic prescribing, the following first-aid advice will be helpful:

• Minor first degree burns may be treated at home. If a

second degree burn has caused minor damage, it may also be appropriate to deal with it using self-help measures. However, if a burn is large (covering an area larger than the size of a two-pence piece), or if a third degree burn has been sustained, **always get professional help as quickly as possible**.
- For straightforward burns, cool the area by immersing it in cool water, or run cold water over the skin.
- Avoid breaking blisters which can lead to an infected wound. If spontaneous breaking of a blister has occurred, bathe the area with Calendula lotion or diluted Hypericum and Calendula tincture to inhibit infection.
- Do not attempt to remove any clothing from a third degree burn. Having sent for medical help as soon as possible, give as much reassurance as you can. If any signs of shock develop, check the appropriate table for possible remedies.

When to seek medical advice
If any of the following occur, get professional help:

- Third degree burns.
- Signs of **shock** including:
  - Confusion or unconsciousness
  - Irregular or shallow breathing
  - Coldness and pallor.
- Indications of infection around the burn including redness, swelling or pus.

There are basic, common-sense steps you can take to try to prevent burns occurring. Although they are not infallible, they can help to protect your child against the possibility of some dangerous burns and scalds occurring.

These include:

- Keeping small children out of the kitchen when meals are being prepared.
- Turning handles of pots and pans away from the edge of your stove so that your child cannot tip the contents over themselves.
- Shortening flexes of electric kettles so that they cannot be reached easily by small hands.
- Making sure that you keep household water temperatures well beneath boiling point: **always** test the temperature of your child's bath water before he goes in, and ensure that central heating radiators are kept at a temperature where they will not burn if a child falls against them.
- Checking that mugs containing very hot drinks are out of reach of a small child, or cats or dogs that could knock them over.
- Locking household cleaners, caustic substances and any other dangerous chemicals away, or placing on sufficiently high shelves that your child cannot reach.

Shock

TYPE	GENERAL INDICATIONS	WORSE FROM	BETTER FOR	REMEDY NAME
Shock with general trauma following an accident or injury	Needed immediately after physical injury with bruising. Swelling, bruised pain, and possible injury to head and neck would suggest the need for this remedy.	Being helped and comforted. Touch	Lying with head lower than the body	Arnica

TYPE	GENERAL INDICATIONS	WORSE FROM	BETTER FOR	REMEDY NAME
Shock with associated fear and restlessness	Shock after physical or emotional trauma with pain and terror. Rapid breathing and palpitations with heightened anxiety state. Sweating with marked trembling.	Chill. Noise. Light	Rest. Open air	Aconite
Shock with state of near-collapse	Strong desire for fresh air or being fanned, which is relieving. Skin feels cold and clammy, and looks very pale. States of severe shock with shallow breathing and bluish tinge to the skin.	Pressure of clothes. Warmth. Lack of fresh air	Cool, fresh air. Being fanned. Elevating feet	Carbo veg

When to seek medical advice

If your child has entered a state of shock, **send for help as quickly as possible**. While you are waiting, consider the following additional advice:

- Give as much reassurance as possible.
- Loosen clothing at neck, waist and chest.
- Avoid exposure to extreme changes from heat to cold.
- Never move your child if you suspect a serious injury has occurred.
- Raise the legs slightly higher than the chest.

Insect bites and stings

TYPE	GENERAL INDICATIONS	WORSE FROM	BETTER FOR	REMEDY NAME
Bites and stings that feel better for cold bathing	Affected area feels cold to the touch and looks very red and swollen. Stinging, pricking pains are made much easier by cold compresses and bathing.	Warmth	Cold	Ledum
Very puffy, pink, hot swelling around site of bite or sting	Strong adverse reaction to heat in any form. Lots of localised pain, heat, redness and swelling which are greatly relieved by cold. Indicated for hives that follow a sting or bite.	Heat. Touch	Cool in any form	Apis
Large, irritating midge bites	Exquisite, stinging, smarting pains with bites. Maddened and extremely irritated both physically and mentally by discomfort.	Touch	Rest. Warmth	Staphysagria
Hives which develop after a sting	Raised red blotches which sting and burn severely. Itching of skin is extremely intense and distressing.	Bathing with cold water. Touch		Urtica urens

General advice

In addition to homoeopathic prescribing after removing the sting, reassure your child and apply cold compresses.

- The sting can be removed with a pair of tweezers held close to the skin. You will need someone to help hold your child and comfort them, since they are likely to be very frightened and in pain. Remember that wasps do not leave a sting behind.
- Avoid squeezing a sting out: this only serves to force the toxin in the sting further into the skin.
- Use diluted Urtica urens tincture to bathe the area affected by the sting, as well as giving a homoeopathic remedy internally.

When to seek medical advice
If any of the following occur, seek professional help immediately:

- If you know your child has an allergic reaction to wasp or bee stings, give Apis 30c and send for help immediately. Signs of an allergic reaction include:
  - Pale or greyish looking skin
  - Cold, clammy skin
  - Weak or fast pulse
  - Gasping or yawning
  - Drowsiness or unconsciousness

  If this situation occurs, it is a **severe medical emergency** and no time should be wasted in getting medical help.
- If your child has been stung in the mouth send for help immediately. If your child is fully conscious try to get her

to sip iced water, or suck on an ice cube. **Do not** give
your child anything to drink if she has lost consciousness.
• Any sign of rapidly-advancing swelling around the mouth
or in the throat.

Dental work

TYPE	GENERAL INDICATIONS	WORSE FROM	BETTER FOR	REMEDY NAME
Anxiety about going to the dentist	State of terror and anguish builds as the time of appointment comes near. Very restless, fearful and desperate with trembling. Specific fear of, and intolerance to, pain	At night	Resting	Aconite
Bruised pain and general trauma following dental work	The first remedy to think of where the mouth is generally sore and painful following procedures such as drilling. If bleeding is scanty following an extraction, select a remedy to speed up healing other than Arnica	Touch		Arnica
Nerve pains caused by drilling or extraction	Pains are characteristically shooting and violent, and radiate from the injured area. Helpful where pain travels from site of injected anaesthetic.	Cold. Touch	Bending head back	Hypericum

TYPE	GENERAL INDICATIONS	WORSE FROM	BETTER FOR	REMEDY NAME
Pains caused by entry of injection	Localised swelling and redness where needle was inserted. Pains are stinging and pricking and considerably relieved by contact with cold. Affected area may also feel cold to the touch.	Warmth	Cold applicat-ions and bathing	Ledum
Pains following drilling or extraction with irritability and hypersensitivity	Snappy, bad-tempered and irritable with pains. Very sensitive to cold: just wants to be warm, quiet and left alone to sleep.	Cold. Touch. Stimulation	A quiet nap. Warmth	Nux vomica
Deep, aching, bruised pain that has not been resolved by Arnica	Pains are located deep in bony tissue which feels bruised. Indicated where bleeding has been too slight following extraction, and a dry socket has occurred. Most helpful in later stages following dental work.	Cold	Warmth	Ruta
Nausea or vomiting after anaesthetic or excessive bleeding	Anxiety with vomiting or bleeding. Relieved by reassurance and comfort. Wants cold drinks, but vomits them back up once they are warmed by the stomach. Copious bleeding from a small wound.	Exertion. Warm food or drink	Affection. Massage. Cold drinks	Phosphorus

TYPE	GENERAL INDICATIONS	WORSE FROM	BETTER FOR	REMEDY NAME
Sharp, stitching, severe pains following dental work	Often needed after extractions: especially where the skin has been cut. Pains are stinging, smarting and sharp. Feelings of anger and resentment following visit to the dentist.	Cold drinks. Touch	Warmth. Rest	Staphysagria

General advice

In addition to homoeopathic prescribing, the following advice will be helpful:

- Try to take the anxiety out of a visit to the dentist by explaining as much as possible about what happens on a routine visit as calmly as you can to your child.
- Stay with your child while treatment is being carried out. You will know what form of reassurance your child will respond to best. This could vary from verbal reassurance, to holding hands, or having a favourite cuddly toy nearby.
- If your child feels off-colour after dental work, give him enough time to recover before going back to school: above all, don't force any activities that seem demanding or tiring too soon.
- If you have doubts about the time it is taking for your child's mouth to heal, or if pain is continuing longer than expected, ring your dentist for advice.
- To speed up healing and to provide a soothing mouthwash, dilute 40 drops of Calendula or Hypericum

and Calendula tincture in $\frac{1}{4}$ pint of cooled, boiled water and get your child to rinse her mouth every few hours for a couple of days. This will also help discourage infection.

CHAPTER 4

CHILDHOOD INFECTIOUS ILLNESSES

Homoeopathic treatment has a very positive role to play in the management of childhood illnesses such as mumps, chicken-pox and measles. While conventional medicine has little to offer in these situations apart from judicious use of painkillers and soothing lotions, skilled homoeopathic prescribing can speed your child through the stages of illness with the minimum amount of distress and complications. High fever, generalised discomfort and itching are all symptoms that can be relieved by the appropriate homoeopathic remedy. Tremendous relief from the distress of itching skin can also be obtained from applying homoeopathic lotions, creams, ointments or diluted tinctures directly to the skin, as well as giving the appropriate remedy internally.

Because homoeopathic medicines work by stimulating the body's own defences to deal more efficiently with disease, rather than attempting to find the specific antidote which will attack the invading organism, childhood infectious illnesses do not pose a greater problem than any other illness to the homoeopath. Within this context we can see that appropriately prescribed homoeopathic medicines are not subject to the same limitations as conventional medicines, because they encourage the body to fight infection irrespective of whether it is viral or bacterial in origin.

The controversy over vaccination

Vaccination is one of the methods employed by conventional medicine in an attempt to control the spread and virulence of childhood diseases. Although sound nutrition and good nursing are also viewed as important in aiding children to fight infectious illnesses, vaccination is portrayed by orthodox practitioners as the main factor which prevents serious complications in small children.

It is not possible within the scope of this chapter to enter into a detailed discussion of the pros and cons of vaccination. However, it is important for parents to realise that there are arguments which suggest that there may be drawbacks to vaccination, beyond the most distressingly obvious such as the controversy over possible neurological damage. Apart from the issues of whether vaccination is effective or not in giving long-term immunity, or the unquestionable historical fact that immunisation played a relatively small role in eliminating infectious diseases, there are other questions relating to the difference between naturally-acquired immunity and an immune response activated by vaccination. Many homoeopaths believe that the latter may lead to long-term problems in children such as recurrent ear infections, skin eruptions and allergic reactions.

Because the issue of vaccination is fraught with anxiety, guilt and confusion, it is essential that you have access to as much factual material as possible in order to make your decision. There are some excellent books available which will give you basic material to work from, as well as organisations such as 'The Informed Parent' who can supply you with information and support through other members.

If you consult a homoeopath about your child, I would

suggest you discuss the issue with them in detail, especially regarding the support they can offer you should your child develop an infectious childhood illness. It is also essential, once you have enough material at your disposal, to discuss the pros and cons of vaccination with your family doctor and health visitor.

For a basic list of publications on this subject, please see the **Further Reading** section at the back of this book.

How to select the appropriate homoeopathic medicine

If you have turned to this section of the book because your child is suffering from the early stages of chicken-pox, this is how you find out which remedy is going to be most helpful.

- Turn to the table entitled **Chicken-pox**, and look down the left hand column entitled *Type* to identify which category your child's symptoms fall into. If your child is hot and flushed with a raised temperature, the chances are that 'Chicken-pox with flushed, hot, red skin and raised temperature' is likely to be the most appropriate.

- Check with the General indications that these symptoms fit with your child's. If her skin is bright red, hot and dry, and if she also has difficulty sleeping, the chances are that you are moving in the right direction. If not, consider other possibilities.

- Check the *Worse from* and *Better for* columns to see

if these also fit. Remember that these columns do not just refer to what makes the specific symptoms of infection better or worse, but also what might make her feel generally better or worse. So if you have noticed that she is much better if she can rest undisturbed, but is very sensitive to any stimulation such as noise and bright light, the chances are that Belladonna will be most suitable.

• Check with the **Keynotes** at the back of the book that the homoeopathic remedy you have selected covers the bulk of your child's symptoms well. Don't worry if all the symptoms mentioned in connection with Belladonna are not presented by your child: remember that you are looking for the closest approximation to the overall symptom picture that she presents. What you need are some major symptoms to work with: in other words, you would not give Belladonna to a child who did not exhibit sudden onset of heat, restlessness, feverishness and high temperature, but who looked pale, droopy and withdrawn, and who complained of feeling achey, shivery and feverish over a gradual period of time. In the latter situation, it is likely that a remedy such as Gelsemium will match the symptoms more closely, since it is very often indicated in slow-developing 'flu-like states.

For information on how to administer the appropriate remedy, see the section entitled *Giving homoeopathic medicines to children* in Chapter 2; exactly the same principles apply.

Mumps

TYPE	GENERAL INDICATIONS	WORSE FROM	BETTER FOR	REMEDY NAME
Rapid onset of symptoms with high temperature and dry skin	Most helpful in early stage of illness. Very feverish with dry skin that radiates heat. Glands look red and inflamed and very sensitive to touch. Dry, sore throat with difficulty swallowing: must sit forward to drink. Not usually thirsty. Throbbing headache with shooting glandular pain.	Touch or slightest pressure. Cold air. Right side. Stooping. Light. Noise	Rest. Warm rooms. Sitting propped-up in bed	Belladonna
Early stage with marked anxiety and restlessness	Sudden onset of violent symptoms. Normally calm child becomes frantic and fearful with fever and pains. Symptoms get worse as night approaches. Pains worse by uncovering or exposure to cold. Thirsty with fever.	Lying on painful side. Approach of night. Exposure to cold	Fresh air. Rest	Aconite
Marked glandular puffiness and swelling with marked heat sensitivity	Rosy-red, puffy swellings including eyelids. Severe, stinging pains made much worse by exposure to heat, and relieved by cold. Constantly fidgety and restless with illness.	Lying down. After sleep. Warmth	Cold. Cool air. Changing position	Apis

TYPE	GENERAL INDICATIONS	WORSE FROM	BETTER FOR	REMEDY NAME
Symptoms which are made worse by slightest movement	Slow, insidious development of symptoms. Lethargic, irritable and antisocial: wants to be left alone. Extreme sensitivity to slightest movement. Headache and constipation with glandular swelling. Dry lips with marked thirst for cold drinks.	Heat. Making an effort. Motion	Keeping still. Perspiring. Cold drinks	Bryonia
Pains which are left-sided or move from left to right	Constricting and throbbing glandular pains which are worse after sleep. Strong aversion to neck being touched or constricted by clothing. Extreme pain and swelling in left-side glands. Swallowing very difficult and painful	Left side. Waking from sleep. Touch. Pressure of clothes around neck. Empty swallow-ing	Swallowing food. Cold drinks. Fresh air	Lachesis
Pressing and tense pains in glands which feel hard	Very painful, stony swellings in glands under the jaw and neck to the ear lobe. Difficulty swallowing with dryness in throat: pains shoot to the ears. Paleness of face with illness.	Night. Warmth of bed. Cold and damp. Swallowing	Warmth in general	Phytolacca

TYPE	GENERAL INDICATIONS	WORSE FROM	BETTER FOR	REMEDY NAME
Weakness and perspiration with illness	Swollen tonsils and stiffness of jaw with glandular swelling. Dryness at back of the throat with marked increase of saliva in mouth. Difficulty in speaking with swelling of glands. Thirsty with flushed, sweaty face.	Cold. After sweating. Left side		Jaborandi
Mumps with bad breath and copious saliva and sweat	All symptoms are worse as the night goes on. Characteristic sweet, unpleasant, metallic taste in the mouth with offensive breath and swollen, enlarged tongue. Most useful in later stage of infection after fever has peaked.	Changes of warmth or cold. Draughts. Sweating. Night	Rest. Even temperatures	Merc sol
Extreme restlessness at night with marked sensitivity to cold and damp	Severe swelling of glands, often worse on left side. Despondency and depression at night with restlessness from aching in limbs. Cold sores may appear on the lips while ill. Very much worse from exposure to cold in any form.	Damp and cold. Night. Keeping still	Warmth. Being wrapped up. Bathing in warm water. Limited movement which does not exhaust	Rhus tox

TYPE	GENERAL INDICATIONS	WORSE FROM	BETTER FOR	REMEDY NAME
Established symptoms which linger with sensitivity to heat	Lingering symptoms with weepiness and need for sympathy. Child may be whiny and in need of a lot of attention. Dry mouth with coated tongue, but no thirst. Much worse for being warm; better for cool surroundings.	Stuffy rooms. Lying down. Night. Warmth in general	Cool, fresh air. Gentle movement. Sympathy and attention	Pulsatilla.

General advice

The following advice will be helpful in addition to homoeopathic prescribing:

- Although you should encourage your child to drink as much as possible when ill, avoid giving acid drinks such as orange juice which make the pain of mumps worse by increasing the flow of saliva. Oranges, lemon juice and spicy food should be avoided, as well as any sweets that have a 'sharp' or acid quality, such as sherberts.
- If your child has difficulty opening her mouth, give drinks through a straw.
- If warmth is soothing and eases the pain, apply warm compresses to the painful area. This could be a warm flannel or a hot water bottle well wrapped in a towel.
- Give foods in the form of soups and purees: these are less effort to eat and easier to digest.
- Keep children in the contagious stage of mumps away from adults who have not contracted the disease, since

the complications in adults can be very unpleasant. These include painful swelling of the testicles and swelling and inflammation of the ovaries and breasts.

When to seek medical advice
If any of the following occur, get professional advice:

- Diminished hearing or vision.
- Stiff neck with headache, weakness or convulsions.
- Pains in the abdomen, especially if accompanied by vomiting.

Measles

TYPE	GENERAL INDICATIONS	WORSE FROM	BETTER FOR	REMEDY NAME
Early stage of illness with marked restlessness and anxiety	Sudden, violent onset of symptoms. Symptoms emerge or get worse as night goes on. Terrible fear and sensitivity to pain. Nasal discharge with very light-sensitive, red eyes. Cough sounds hard and croupy. Skin burns and itches.	Warmth. Night	Open air	Aconite

TYPE	GENERAL INDICATIONS	WORSE FROM	BETTER FOR	REMEDY NAME
Early stage of illness with rapid rise in temperature and very dry, hot skin	Symptoms develop with violence and rapidity. Skin bright red and dry with fever, radiating heat. Very drowsy, and irritable but can't sleep. Rapid pulse with restlessness and throbbing headache. Sticking pains with sore throat causing distress when drinking.	Stimulation. Light. Noise. Cold air	Lying quietly semi-erect in bed. Warm rooms	Belladonna
Measles with puffy swelling of face, eyes and eyelids	Rash appears slowly with stinging pains that are relieved by cold bathing. Heat causes distress in any form. Rash is rosy pink, puffy and very itchy making child very fidgety. Eyelids may look like 'water bags'.	Heat. Touch. After sleep	Cold bathing. Cool air. Being on the move	Apis.
Slow developing symptoms with great lethargy and weariness	Insidious development of illness. Alternating fever and high temperature with chills, aching and shivering. Red, puffy face with drooping eyelids. Drowsy, lethargic and apathetic: wants to be left alone.	Effort of any kind	Open air. Passing water. Warmth	Gelsemium

TYPE	GENERAL INDICATIONS	WORSE FROM	BETTER FOR	REMEDY NAME
Measles with distressing eye symptoms	Light sensitivity with streaming, burning, painful watering from the eyes. Nasal discharge is bland. Nose and eye symptoms are better for open air. Hoarseness with dry cough.	Evening. Light. Warmth	Open air. Blinking or wiping eyes	Euphrasia
Established stage of illness when fever has peaked and rash has come out	Dry mouth with no thirst. Alternating dry and loose cough: dry at night and loose on waking. Bland, thick and greenish-yellow discharges. Weepy and clingy with illness. Rash aggravated by warmth.	Rest. Warmth. Stuffy rooms. Eating	Gentle motion. Cool, fresh air. Cool bathing. Sympathy	Pulsatilla
Slow-developing symptoms with severe cough	Painful, dry, chesty cough from irritation and tickling in larynx. Intense thirst for cold drinks with dry mouth. Movement aggravates symptoms: headache worse from coughing. Irritable and constipated with illness.	Movement. Becoming hot. Eating. Sitting up	Quiet. Rest. Cool, open air. Cold drinks. Firm pressure	Bryonia

General advice

The following advice will be helpful in addition to homoeopathic prescribing:

- If your child is very light-sensitive, make sure that you keep exposure to light to a minimum by dimming lights and drawing curtains.
- Do not force food on your child if he is not hungry, especially in the feverish stage. However, do make sure that your child drinks as much as possible, in order to guard against dehydration. When your child wants to eat, keep meals as light and digestible as possible.
- Avoid heavy, indigestible foods and try to introduce soups, broths or purées.

When to seek medical advice
If any of the following occur, get professional advice:

- Breathing difficulties.
- Persistently high temperature with distress or lethargy.
- Severe headache with vomiting.
- Eye infection.
- Measles in a child under six months of age.
- Persistent cough which refuses to clear up with self-help measures.
- Fever which doesn't resolve itself when the rash comes out.
- Bleeding from orifices or under the skin.

Chicken-pox

TYPE	GENERAL INDICATIONS	WORSE FROM	BETTER FOR	REMEDY NAME
Dry, hot, bright red skin with sudden onset of fever	Violent and abrupt onset of symptoms. Feverishness and rapid pulse with throbbing headache which prevents sleep. Very bad-tempered and sensitive to disturbance. Skin feels very hot and dry and looks flushed except for pale area around mouth.	Bright light. Noise. Being disturbed. Exposure to cold	Lying propped up in bed. Resting undisturbed	Belladonna
Early stage of illness with fever and marked restlessness	Symptoms develop rapidly with distressing anxiety accompanying fever. Thirst with feverishness, but no perspiration. Screams and panics with discomfort and anxiety.	As night goes on. Warm rooms. Exposure to chill	Fresh air. Sleep. After perspiring	Aconite
Chicken-pox with marked chilliness and restlessness	Very anxious with illness: needs a lot of reassurance and company. Burning and itching that is relieved by warmth, worse from being cold. Large eruptions which look pussy. Very distressed with approach of night.	Effort. Cold. Being alone. At night	Warmth. Sips of warm drinks. Lying propped-up in bed	Arsenicum album

TYPE	GENERAL INDICATIONS	WORSE FROM	BETTER FOR	REMEDY NAME
Rash which is very itchy and worse from exposure to cold	Very restless and desperate with symptoms, especially in bed at night. Cannot get to sleep because of itching. More despondent and depressed than anxious. Itching is relieved by warm bathing.	Scratching. In bed. At night. Exposure to cold	Moderate temperatures. Warm bathing	Rhus tox
Slow-developing rash with chesty cough	Rattling cough with rash that emerges slowly. Skin feels cold and eruptions are large with a bluish tinge. Itching is worse after bathing or from warmth of bed. Tongue is coated with thick white fur. Very bad-tempered with onset of illness.	Exposure to water. In the evening. Lying down.	Cool air. Bringing up phlegm	Ant tart
Swollen glands with chicken-pox and heavy perspiration	Bad breath and offensive sweat with illness. Bad taste in the mouth that is metallic or sweet-tasting with increased saliva. Large eruptions with a lot of pus that develop into sores. Indicated in later stages of illness.	Heat. Cold. As night goes on	Resting in even temperature	Merc sol

TYPE	GENERAL INDICATIONS	WORSE FROM	BETTER FOR	REMEDY NAME
Low-grade fever with weepiness and clinginess	Useful in established stage of illness. Swollen glands with lingering unresolved fever. Child demands attention and responds well when it is given. Dry mouth with no thirst; chilliness with aversion to warmth.	Warmth. Resting. At night. Stuffy, airless rooms	Cool, fresh, open air. Attention and sympathy. Cool bathing. Gentle motion	Pulsatilla

General advice

The following advice will be helpful in addition to homoeopathic prescribing:

- Trim your child's nails as short as possible to prevent blisters being broken. This will help to prevent infection or scarring.
- When the blisters have reached the crusty stage, avoid rubbing them with a towel after bathing but pat them dry gently to avoid damaging the scabs.
- Avoid putting your child in a hot bath as the rash is emerging: this can be very enervating and make the rash more irritable.
- If the skin is very itchy once the rash has come out, an oatmeal bath can be very soothing. Alternatively you can add Hypericum and Calendula or Urtica urens tincture to your child's bathwater, or soak cotton wool pads with either diluted tincture and bathe the rash as often as possible.
- Avoid giving aspirin to bring down a fever since it may be

implicated in the development of Reye's syndrome. This is a serious illness characterised by high temperature, vomiting and kidney and liver problems.

- While your child is not hungry don't feel compelled to offer or force food on him. Make sure drinks are given often, and once your child is hungry offer meals that are as light and easily digestible as possible.

When to seek medical advice
If any of the following occur, professional help is needed:

- Infected skin eruption, very severe itching, or bleeding under the skin.
- Chicken-pox in a child under one year of age.
- Rapid, shallow breathing or vomiting.
- Severe headache, stiff neck, convulsions and persistent lethargy or weakness.
- If spots affect the eyes.

Whooping cough

TYPE	GENERAL INDICATIONS	WORSE FROM	BETTER FOR	REMEDY NAME
Bouts of coughing with cold, clammy sweat	Initially red with coughing bout, then very pale, cold and clammy. Raw feeling in throat with burning sensation in chest. 'Air hunger' with desire for cool, fresh air. Cough initially hard and dry, followed by lots of mucus.	Warmth. Walking. Night	Being fanned. Cool, open air	Carbo veg

TYPE	GENERAL INDICATIONS	WORSE FROM	BETTER FOR	REMEDY NAME
Metallic, dry cough with hoarseness	Severe, violent bouts of coughing that follow each other in quick succession. Cough begins as soon as child lies down. Barking cough comes from deep in abdomen.	Drinking. Lying down. Talking or laughing. Warmth	Open air. Activity	Drosera
Coughing bouts that are worse for stuffy rooms	Coughing begins while trying to clear throat of mucus. Needs to swallow constantly. Bout of coughing ends with vomiting stringy, difficult to move mucus which hangs from mouth.	Warmth. Stuffy rooms	Sips of water. Cool room	Coccus cacti
Wheezy, rattling cough with gagging	Child may stiffen during a coughing spasm and briefly lose breath. Skin may look bluish during coughing bout. Cough ends in gagging and vomiting. All symptoms are much worse for movement. Nose bleeds may accompany cough.	Movement. Lying down. Damp air	Rest. Open air. Cold drinks	Ipecac

TYPE	GENERAL INDICATIONS	WORSE FROM	BETTER FOR	REMEDY NAME
Whooping cough with easy bringing up of mucus	Sensitive feeling in chest during bouts of coughing. Dry, barking cough in cold air, becoming loose in warm room. Choking sensation followed by vomiting. Must sit forward for relief during spasms.	Draughts. Cold. Lying down. After exertion	Moderate temperatures. During the day. Moving about	Kali carb
Smothering sensations precede bouts of coughing	Dry cough with profuse nasal catarrh. Stringy mucus is vomited up after coughing spasms. Too cold when uncovered, and too hot when covered. Bouts of coughing in rapid succession.	Inhaling air. Eating. Change of air	Heat	Corallium rubrum
Sore, aching and bruised sensations in chest with coughing	Cough worse during sleep and exercise. Cries out before cough begins anticipating pain it brings. Holds chest when coughing to minimise pain.	Exertion. Damp cold. At night	Resting	Arnica

General advice

In addition to homoeopathic prescribing, the following advice may be helpful:

- See the general advice in the *Cough* section of the chapter on **Acute Problems in Infants and Children**.

Although not specifically relating to whooping cough, it will still prove useful in providing general advice on how to make your child more comfortable.

- Reassure your child as much as possible during coughing spasms by talking calmly, stroking or holding them. The coughing spasms associated with whooping cough can be very alarming for both parent and child, but anxiety and panic will make it even harder for your child to breathe.
- Babies can be assisted in coughing bouts by holding them face down across your knees with their backs toward you. Older children can be helped by encouraging them to lean forward in a sitting position.
- Give drinks and small meals just after a coughing bout so that your child has a better chance of keeping them down. Anything eaten or drunk just before a coughing spasm is likely to be vomited up.
- Make sure your child does not get dehydrated by encouraging him to drink as much fluid as possible. This is very important if vomiting is happening on a regular basis over an extended period of time.

When to seek medical advice
If any of the following occur, get professional help:

- Whooping cough in children is a particularly serious illness. If you suspect the onset of symptoms, notify your health practitioner, and, if necessary, arrange for an examination in order to confirm diagnosis.
- Whooping cough in a baby, especially under six months of age.
- Wheezing or accelerated breathing in between coughing bouts.
- Marked chest pain.

- Headache, confusion or drowsiness.
- If symptoms are not responding to self-help measures and you suspect your child's health is declining rather than improving.

German measles

TYPE	GENERAL INDICATIONS	WORSE FROM	BETTER FOR	REMEDY NAME
Sudden onset of symptoms with restlessness before rash has come out	Very distressed and anxious with rapid onset of illness. Runny nose with red, sensitive eyes. Sleep is restless and fitful with aggravation of symptoms at night. Dry, croupy cough with possible diarrhoea. Thirsty with fever.	Warm rooms. At night. Light	Resting. Sleep	Aconite
Early stage of symptoms with high fever and very dry, red skin	Red face with throbbing headache. Rapid pulse with high temperature. Drowsy and frustrated because discomfort prevents sleep. Over-sensitive to any stimulation. Limbs twitch and jerk in fitful sleep.	Light. Noise. Jarring. Motion	Lying semi-propped up in bed. Darkened rooms	Belladonna
Early stage of illness with less rapid or violent onset than Aconite or Belladonna	Flushed and hot with fever, with red patches on cheeks. Easily tired, but more alert with fever than Belladonna and less anxious than Aconite.	At night. Cold. Making an effort	Warmth. Cold applications	Ferrum phos

TYPE	GENERAL INDICATIONS	WORSE FROM	BETTER FOR	REMEDY NAME
Later stage of illness with swollen glands and congested sinuses	Indicated when the fever has subsided and child is left with rattly cough and obstructed nose. Mucus is thick, yellow and stringy and causes pain and pressure at the root of the nose. Indifferent and apathetic with illness.	Exposure to cold. Undressing. Early hours of the morning	Warmth. Firm pressure	Kali bich
Established stage of illness with eye or ear problems that linger	All discharges are thick, bland and yellowish-green. Ear and gland pains that are worse from warmth and better for cool conditions. Dry mouth with no thirst. Restlessness, weepiness and need for sympathy and attention.	Resting. Warmth. Stuffy rooms. At night. Rich or fatty foods	Gentle motion. Cool, fresh air. Sympathy and comfort. Cool applications	Pulsatilla

General Advice

See general advice given in *Measles* section and the indications which require professional advice. Since German measles tends to be a much milder illness than other childhood infectious diseases, you may not need to give a homoeopathic remedy if your child is coping very well on her own.

- Remember that you should prevent any woman who is pregnant coming in contact with a child who has German measles. You should also contact any pregnant women who may have been in the company of your child during the incubation period of the illness (three weeks before the rash came out).

CHAPTER 5

PROBLEMS IN BABIES AND INFANTS

You will find conditions included in this chapter that are especially relevant to babies. However, other problems that occur in babyhood can also be found in other appropriate sections, e.g. vomiting and diarrhoea in the chapter on **Acute Problems**, or chicken-pox under **Childhood Infectious Diseases**. To get the maximum help from these sections, combine the information contained in them as creatively as you wish. For example, if your baby has a sore throat with a cold and cough, you can use the relevant information included in all three tables (which can be found in **Acute Problems**) in order to decide which is the most appropriate homoeopathic remedy for your baby.

A note on dosage for babies

Do not be misled into thinking that babies need a different method of administering their appropriate homoeopathic remedy because they are so young. Unlike orthodox medicines where dosage is normally reduced to accommodate the age of a patient, homoeopathic remedies are given in the same way to babies and children as to adults.

Because babies cannot cooperate by sucking a tablet, it is best to crush the selected homoeopathic remedy between two clean spoons. Take a pinch of this fine powder and rub it along your baby's gums, or place a small amount in the area where the gum and cheek meet. Older children will suck on homoeopathic tablets very happily until they are dissolved; this is due to the milk sugar base of the tablets which makes them taste appetising to children.

Homoeopathic remedies are not only obtainable in tablet form: you can order remedies in granules, globules or liquids in dropper bottles from homoeopathic pharmacies. You can also buy creams, ointments, tinctures and lotions from the same source.

Taking note of your baby's symptoms

Because your baby cannot speak to you and answer relevant questions, it is clear that you need to rely on other skills in order to put together a useful symptom picture of your baby's illness. Your powers of observation will provide you with the bulk of information that you need. The following are some suggestions of questions you might want to ask yourself:

How does the appearance of my baby differ from normal?
Is she more flushed, pale, sweaty, hot or dry than usual?
Is she restless, withdrawn, anxious, or more irritable than usual?
Does she want to be comforted more than usual?
Has there been a precipitating factor such as a chill, shock, or accident before the symptoms emerged?

Have there been any changes in her average sleeping or feeding
   pattern?
Is she constipated, or does she have diarrhoea?
Has she had any spots, rashes, or changes in skin texture?
How does she react to fresh air or warmth?
How does she react to noise or light?

You can work from this basic list adding any other questions
that strike you as relevant. Follow your instincts and
remember you are interested in any changes from what is
normal for your baby. In other words, if your baby is pale by
nature this is not a relevant symptom for acute prescribing.
However, if your usually pale child looks very flushed, this is
important because it indicates a change from what is normal.

A note of caution

It is always worth bearing in mind that illness can develop
rapidly in babies and children. For this reason, if you
suspect that your baby may be seriously ill always seek
medical help as quickly as possible.

How to select the appropriate homoeopathic medicine

If you have turned to this section of the book because your
baby is very distressed with teething pains, this is how you
select the appropriate homoeopathic remedy:

• Turn to the table entitled **Teething** and look down the left hand column entitled *Type* to identify which category your baby's symptoms fall into. If your baby is normally placid and even-tempered, but since teething has been clingy and very demanding on your sympathy and attention, the chances are that Teething with clinginess and possible catarrhal involvement is a category worth considering.

• Check with the *General Indications* that these symptoms fit with your baby's. If your baby is apathetic rather than frustrated with pain, and especially if he or she is quickly comforted by being given attention and sympathy, it looks like you are moving in the right direction. If, in addition, your baby had also been very stuffed up since teething, this would be a confirmatory symptom; especially if the mucus was yellowy-green in colour.

• Finally check the *Worse from* and *Better for* columns to see if these also fit. Do bear in mind that these do not just apply to the factors that make the teething symptoms better or worse, but also what might make your baby generally better or worse. So, if you have noticed that your baby responds well to being carried out of doors in the fresh open air, but seems to be worse for resting in a warm environment, the chances are that you have found the appropriate remedy.

• Turn to the **Keynotes** section at the back of the book to confirm your choice. Don't worry if all the symptoms mentioned in connection with the remedy are not present in your baby; remember that what you are looking for is the closest approximation to the overall picture presented by him or her. What you need are some essential symptoms to work with: in other words, you would not give Pulsatilla to a baby who reacted badly to sympathy and attention, or cool fresh air, who felt better in warm surroundings.

For information on how to administer the appropriate remedy, in addition to *A Note on Dosage for Babies* above, see the section entitled *Giving homoeopathic remedies to children* Chapter 2; exactly the same principles apply.

Teething

TYPE	GENERAL INDICATIONS	WORSE FROM	BETTER FOR	REMEDY NAME
Irritability with teething in an otherwise calm baby.	Restlessness and whining: nothing seems to please or pacify. Slightly feverish with teething, with possible diarrhoea. One cheek may be flushed while the other is pale and cool. May toss about and cry out suddenly in sleep.	Draughts. Exposure to wind. In the first part of the night	Being rocked, carried, or driven in a car	Chamomilla
Teething with red, flushed face	Baby may strike out or bite with irritability. Skin is bright red, very hot and dry to the touch. Senses may be over-acute, starting at the least touch, noise or jolt. Very restless sleep with a tendency to jerk awake.	Bright light. Noise	Warm wraps. Warm room	Belladonna

TYPE	GENERAL INDICATIONS	WORSE FROM	BETTER FOR	REMEDY NAME
Teething with screaming and anxiety	Terrific restlessness in a baby who looks frightened. Easily startled, with an aversion to being touched or uncovered. May be feverish with hot head and a cool body.	Extremes of temperature. Warm rooms. Exposure to cold winds	Open air. After sleep	Aconite
Teething with diarrhoea and lots of wind	Often indicated for children who are late in teething and slow in learning to walk. Delayed development may be accompanied by difficulties in assimilating nutrients from food.	Movement. Exertion	Resting. Hot bathing	Calc phos
Teething with clinginess and possible catarrhal involvement	Baby seems very clingy and pathetic with pain, and responds well to sympathy and being distracted. If catarrh is present it will be persistent, green, thick and bland. May be very stuffed up at night with lots of loud breathing through the mouth.	Being still. Warmth. Being in a stuffy room	Sympathy. Fresh air. Cool, dry air, drinks, or food.	Pulsatilla

TYPE	GENERAL INDICATIONS	WORSE FROM	BETTER FOR	REMEDY NAME
Teething with bad breath	Restlessness and irritability with pains. Hot face with cold legs and feet. May be drowsy all day and restless all night. Gums are very inflamed and bleed easily: may look 'spongy'. When teeth come through they have poor quality enamel and quickly develop cavities.	Out of doors. Lying down. Being touched	Warmth. Warm food. Moving about. Pressure	Kreosotum
Slow, painful, difficult teething with possible accompanying diarrhoea	Teething may occur very much later than the expected time. Other milestones such as closure of fontanelles, crawling and walking may also be a long time in coming. Babies who are normally placid, mild and good-tempered when well become very stubborn and difficult to manage when teething. Sweat and other discharges smell sour.	Exposure to damp and cold. Making an effort. Fresh air. Milk	Being constipated. Warmth. Lying down	

General advice

The following may be helpful in addition to choosing the most appropriate homoeopathic remedy:

- Let your baby bite on a cool teething ring or suck on a clean, cool flannel (it is often helpful to keep it in the fridge before use).
- Because firm pressure is often soothing, try rubbing your baby's gums to relieve discomfort. It is also possible to buy biscuits which are suitable for babies to chew on while teething.
- Try to avoid resorting to sedatives where possible. If the appropriate homoeopathic remedy is administered it should relieve pain and ease distress within a short space of time. If you are having trouble selecting a suitable remedy, or your baby is not responding, consult a professional homoeopath.

Colic

TYPE	GENERAL INDICATIONS	WORSE FROM	BETTER FOR	REMEDY NAME
Colicky pains with skin that is red, hot and dry to the touch	Spasmodic pains that come and go quickly. Lots of irritability with pains and general bad temper. Skin generally, or on the abdomen, may be so flushed and hot that it radiates heat. May bend backwards or forwards to get relief from pain.	Jarring. Stimulation. Pressure or touch	Resting. Warmth	Belladonna

TYPE	GENERAL INDICATIONS	WORSE FROM	BETTER FOR	REMEDY NAME
Pains with extreme irritability and temper	Screams and doubles up with pains that nothing seems to pacify. Throws toys around in fits of temper. Teething and diarrhoea may accompany pains of colic. Bloating of the abdomen is not relieved by passing wind.	At night	Being rocked or carried. Heat locally applied	Chamomilla
Colic with marked bloating of the abdomen, and lots of rumbling and gurgling after eating	Marked bloating and discomfort after every meal, but the worst symptoms come on between 4-8 p.m. Reacts badly to any pressure around the area of discomfort. Problems may come on as a result of breast-feeding mother eating indigestible, overly-fibrous diet.	Pressure. Early afternoon to evening. Cold foods and drinks. Warm rooms. On waking	Open air. Pressure being relieved around abdomen. Passing wind. Warm food or drinks	Lycopodium

TYPE	GENERAL INDICATIONS	WORSE FROM	BETTER FOR	REMEDY NAME
Pains that are very much worse for movement with marked irritability and constipation	Infant feels much better for lying still and firm pressure, but may react badly to light touch. Mucous membranes feel dry and marked thirst is likely to be present. Stubborn constipation. When a stool is eventually passed it is large, hard, dark, dry and crumbly. Draws legs up to abdomen in an effort to get comfortable	Movement. Light touch. Warm rooms. Jarring	Firm pressure. Being still. Open air	Bryonia
Colic which is obviously relieved from pressure	Pains are relieved by doubling-up or by infant lying on stomach, or pressing on the painful area with fists. Stopping the infant from doing this results in protests and crying. Abrupt onset and relief from violent, spasmodic pains.	Keeping still. Release of firm pressure	Heat locally applied. Movement. Passing wind	Colocynthis
Colicky pains that are relieved by warmth .	Pains are relieved by eating, hot water, and warmth. Feels worse if clothing is restrictive or presses on abdomen. There may be a lot of wind, but releasing it does not help. Prostration may accompany the pains.	Exposure to cold. Cold drinks. Touch. At night. Movement	Bending double. Warmth. Firm pressure. Resting	Mag phos

TYPE	GENERAL INDICATIONS	WORSE FROM	BETTER FOR	REMEDY NAME
Colic with fruitless attempts at vomiting or moving bowels	Irritability with colic which is worse after waking from sleep. Gags in attempting to vomit, but nothing comes up. Straining in attempting to empty bowels, but very little, or nothing, is passed. Overall sensitivity on emotional and physical levels, which includes hyper-sensitivity to pain. Colic may follow on from breast-feeding mother having eaten very spicy food, or having an excess of alcohol or coffee.	Cold draughts of air. Disturbed sleep. After eating. Touch	Unbroken sleep. Resting	Nux vomica
Colic with very changeable bowel movements: no two stools look alike	Tearfulness with colicky pains and alternation between diarrhoea and constipation. Symptoms may follow on from breast-feeding mother having too much fatty food, ice-cream or fruit. Infant responds well to cuddles and sympathy	Evenings. Stuffy rooms. Being still. Too many bed covers	Fresh air. Gentle movement. Uncover-ing. Sympathy	Pulsatilla

TYPE	GENERAL INDICATIONS	WORSE FROM	BETTER FOR	REMEDY NAME
Colic in babies with severe, rumbling wind.	Baby arches backwards in order to get relief from pain (the opposite of babies requiring *Chamomilla* who draw their knees up to relieve discomfort of colic). Dislikes lying down and feels better for being held upright	Bending forward. In the morning. Lying down	Arching backward. Stretching out	Dioscorea

General advice

The following advice may also be helpful:

• If you are breast feeding, try to avoid foods that may aggravate colic in your baby. These include:

Alcohol
Tea
Spices
Chocolate
Coffee
Raw peppers

Cabbage, cauliflower and Brussels sprouts
Oranges
Grapes
Eggs and dairy foods in general, including cows' milk

• Check the size of teat on your baby's bottle: if it is too big for a new-born, or too small for an older baby, he or she may be swallowing air with the feed which they can't bring up.
• Check that your baby isn't constipated.
• Help your baby to bring up wind after a feed

When to seek medical advice
If any of the following occur, get professional advice:

- You are concerned by the distress of your baby.
- If there is any sign of pain being accompanied by vomiting, constipation, diarrhoea or diminished flow of urine.
- You observe signs of dehydration:
  Sunken fontanelles (the soft spot at the crown of the head in new-born babies).
  Sunken eyes.
  Dry mouth or eyes.
  Reduced urine output or strong urine.
  Loss of skin tone.

Nappy rash

TYPE	GENERAL INDICATIONS	WORSE FROM	BETTER FOR	REMEDY NAME
Rash which is soothed by warm bathing	Anxiety, restlessness and general prostration if rash is severe. May have digestive disturbance with rash. Chilly and generally relieved for a short time by warmth in any form, even though rash burns.	At night. Cold. Exertion	Warmth. Warm food or drinks. Movement	Arsenicum album

TYPE	GENERAL INDICATIONS	WORSE FROM	BETTER FOR	REMEDY NAME
Nappy rash in large, sweaty, infants with sour-smelling discharges	Rash in infants who are slow to pass through developmental stages such as closure of fontanelles, teething and walking. Subject to easy head sweats at night. Pale with a tendency to gain weight quickly.	Exposure to cold. Effort and exertion. Change of weather	Warmth. When constipated	Calc carb
Rash which looks bright red, irritable, and angry	Terrific irritability in infants whose skin feels very dry and hot; heat may radiate from the surface of the skin. Rash leads to general over-sensitivity of the skin.	Lying on the affected area. Stimulation. Cold. Movement	Rest. Warm rooms	Belladonna
Burning nappy rash which is made worse from the slightest touch	Terrific restlessness that disturbs sleep at night, leaving the infant drowsy through the day. General state of hypersensitivity with pains that are burning in character. Much worse after urinating	Movement. Touch	Cool compresses	Cantharis

TYPE	GENERAL INDICATIONS	WORSE FROM	BETTER FOR	REMEDY NAME
Rash which is very rosy red, shiny, sore and hot	Infant may be very intolerant of heat, and much more comfortable for being cooled by uncovering. Also likely to react very badly to touch because of sensitive nature of skin.	Heat in any form. Touch or pressure. Getting wet	Cool air. Uncovering	Apis
Nappy rash which is much worse at night, and causes marked restlessness	Flaky, itchy, burning rash which is relieved by covering and worse for exposure to cold. Infants want to be carried and generally feel much better for motion provided they don't get exhausted.	Exposure to cold and damp. Draughts. Lying down. At night	Movement. Being covered	Rhus tox
Raw nappy rash that is much worse for bathing	Very itchy rash that looks raw and may bleed. Terrific sensitivity to heat, especially the heat of the bed which makes all the symptoms worse. Also reacts badly to washing.	Heat in any form. Washing or bathing. Stuffy rooms	Uncovering. Fresh air	Sulphur

General advice

The following advice may also be of use:
NB The remedies suggested above are intended for use in the isolated bout of nappy rash. If your infant shows tendencies towards repeated bouts of nappy rash which refuse

to clear, it is a situation that requires help from a professional in order to deal with the underlying imbalance which is causing the problem. Also take care with deep-acting remedies such as Sulphur or Calc carb. These should not be repeated frequently, since they can promote a deep-seated, long-term action where the symptoms agree with those of your infant. If in doubt, wait and see, or consult a professional homoeopath.

- Apart from giving the appropriate homoeopathic remedy internally, Calendula or a combination of Hypericum and Calendula ointment can be very soothing. Apply the ointment after each change of nappy, making sure that the affected area has been thoroughly dried.
- Avoid using plastic pants if your baby has a rash.
- Leave your baby's bottom uncovered for as long as it is practically possible, ensuring that the room is warm enough to avoid a chill.
- Experiment with different types of disposable nappies and liners.
- Avoid fruit juice.
- Eliminate the use of biological powders when washing towelling nappies: use soap powder instead, and make sure that the nappies are thoroughly rinsed.

Thrush

TYPE	GENERAL INDICATIONS	WORSE FROM	BETTER FOR	REMEDY NAME
Itchy genital thrush which is offensive. Oral thrush with lots of saliva	All discharges tend to smell offensive. Genital discharge may be greenish and cause distress because it feels acrid and burning. Breath may smell foul with oral thrush, and the tongue may look flabby and coated.	Being chilled. Over-heating. At night. Touch. After eating	Resting. During the day	Mercurius
Oral thrush causes such distress that baby may refuse to feed	Hot mouth with thrush which may affect tongue and gums. Mouth bleeds easily, and there may be an excess of saliva. Discharge of genital thrush looks like egg white.	Touch. Feeding		Borax
Yellow-streaked discharges with thrush	Tongue may be streaked with yellow in oral thrush, and there may be a yellow-coloured discharge with genital thrush. Mucus discharges may be tenacious and ropy.	At night. Touch. Out of doors. Motion	Rest	Hydrastis

TYPE	GENERAL INDICATIONS	WORSE FROM	BETTER FOR	REMEDY NAME
Oral thrush with dry mucus membranes leading to thirst. Very itchy genital thrush with discharge like egg white	Gums and tongue may be coated white and lips may be so dry that they are sore and crack in the middle. Baby may be much worse for attention and sympathy. Genital discharge may be thick and white, or more watery. Although chilly, may react badly to warm rooms.	Sympathy and attention. Warmth. Sunlight	Resting. Lying down	Natrum mur
Oral thrush with white-coated tongue.	All discharges are characterised by their whiteness. In oral thrush in breast-feeding babies, tongue and gums may be covered with a white coating. Genital thrush is very itchy overnight.	Warmth of bed. Motion		Kali mur

General advice

In addition to homoeopathic prescribing, the following advice may be helpful:

Oral thrush
- Try to keep foods as cool, bland and nutritious as possible; hot or acidic foods can aggravate the pain.
- Give drinks in a bottle or through a straw.
- Make sure you sterilise teats and dummies very carefully.

If you are breast-feeding, wash your nipples thoroughly
(avoiding soap) in order to prevent them being infected.
- Dab a solution of water and cider vinegar inside the
affected area of your baby's mouth. The solution should
be made up of $\frac{1}{4}$ pint of boiled and cooled water to one
teaspoon of vinegar.

Genital thrush
- Leave your baby's nappy off for as long a period as is
practically possible.
- Use live yoghurt as an application around the itchy area.
- Make sure you change nappies frequently and avoid using
soap when you wash the affected area. Also steer clear of
scented bubble baths and talcum powder.
- After washing nappies in non-biological or unscented
soap powder, ensure that they are rinsed thoroughly in
order to prevent residues of soap being left behind.
- Bathe your baby's bottom with a diluted solution of
Hypericum and Calendula tincture. Add half a
teaspoonful to a basin of water. You can also add half a
cup of cider vinegar to your baby's bath water.
- Avoid using the same towels as your baby in an effort to
avoid spreading the infection.

When to seek medical advice
If any of the following occur, get professional advice:

- The thrush does not respond to self-help measures within
a few days.
- If there are any indications of pus formation.

Cradle cap

TYPE	GENERAL INDICATIONS	WORSE FROM	BETTER FOR	REMEDY NAME
Eruption on scalp which is better for warmth	Baby is very sensitive to cold, draughty and wet conditions. Cradle cap will be characteristically flakey and itchy, causing a generally restless state.	Exposure to cold. Damp. Night	Warmth	Rhus tox
Cradle cap with lots of scaling and very sweaty head	There may be an offensive smell to the eruption which is likely to cover the whole scalp with a thick layer of scaling. Sweat may stain the pillow yellow. Child may be chilly and lethargic and restless at night. Skin may be generally dry with a tendency to crack.	Motion. Washing. Warmth of bed. In open air	Resting. Cool applications	Graphites
Cradle cap with brown, crusty, scaly eruptions	Scalp will feel uncomfortable from being covered and better for being uncovered. General dryness of skin texture with tendencies to chapping.	Touch. Being covered. Warm room. Warmth of bed	Movement. Uncover-ing. Open air	Lycopodium

TYPE	GENERAL INDICATIONS	WORSE FROM	BETTER FOR	REMEDY NAME
Cradle cap with sour-smelling head sweat	Baby may be large, pale and chilly with a tendency to sour-smelling discharges. Head may be very sweaty overnight, leaving the pillow damp. May also show tendencies towards constipation.	Cold, damp air. Exposure to sun. Washing	From being touched. Wiping or soothing with hands. Uncovering when over-heated. When constipated	Calc carb
Cradle cap which is very itchy and smelly	Baby cannot tolerate exposure to heat or bathing. All discharges tend to smell offensive. Eruptions may be thick and grey-looking. Baby may get over-heated very quickly.	Warmth of bed. Warm room. Extreme cold. Bathing	Cool air. Open air	Sulphur

General advice

Y ou may not need to consider homoeopathic prescribing since the following measures may be helpful enough on their own if cradle cap is mild:

- Apply Calendula cream or ointment to your baby's scalp in the morning and evening.
- Rub your baby's scalp with almond or olive oil (almond oil has a slightly lighter texture) at night. Comb it gently the following day, helping to detach the scales without pulling. Wash your baby's head with a mild shampoo and rinse thoroughly to ensure no soap remains.
- Avoid picking off the crusts.

When to seek medical advice

If any of the following occur, seek professional advice:

- If the cradle cap is very severe or if there are signs of infection, such as weeping or oozing, beneath the crusts.
- If the area is red, itchy or very sore.
- If there is no response to self-help measures within a few days.

CHAPTER 6

ACUTE PROBLEMS IN INFANTS AND CHILDREN

In this section you will find a range of conditions that can be loosely classed as 'acute'. In other words, they have a limited life span with clearly defined stages, such as the common cold.

Acute problems will generally clear up of their own accord if reasonable conditions are provided to support the body in its fight against infection. These conditions include: reasonable amounts of rest, a stable environment with as little fluctuation in surrounding temperature as possible, and an appropriate diet. The latter may involve withholding food, especially if it is indigestible, and concentrating on fluids. Because of the limited nature of acute problems, do not feel obliged to give your child a homoeopathic remedy if they are coping very well by themselves they may not need homoeopathic prescribing.

If your baby or very small child has developed an acute problem, you will find the information included in the section *Taking Note of Symptoms of Your Baby* in Chapter 5 invaluable in pointing you towards the relevant questions you should ask yourself.

Acute problems tend to respond very well to homoeopathic prescribing, which can often speed up the course of the illness and help guard against complications. However, if complications do occur and you suspect your child is entering a serious phase of illness, always call on professional help.

How to select the appropriate homoeopathic medicine

If you have turned to this section of the book because your child has the initial symptoms of a sore throat, this is how you select the appropriate remedy:

- Turn to the table entitled **Sore throats**, and look down the left-hand column entitled *Type* to identify which category your child's symptoms fall into. If, for example, she had been playing quite happily out of doors on a chilly day, but complained of a sore throat which came on rapidly afterwards, the chances are that the column entitled 'Sore throat brought on by exposure to cold, dry winds' is likely to be most useful.

- Check with the *General Indications* in the next column that the majority of these symptoms fit with those presented by your child. If she is uncharacteristically anxious and distressed out of proportion to the symptoms, is feverish with a hot head and chilly body, and the symptoms have developed quickly and violently, it looks like you are moving in the right direction. Remember that you are looking for the general symptom picture that most snuggly matches your child's.

- Finally, check the *Worse from* and *Better for* columns to see if these also fit. Remember that these two columns do not just refer to what makes your child's throat symptoms feel better or worse, but also what makes her generally feel better or worse. So, if, for example, you have definitely noticed that she feels worse as the night goes on, and from being in a warm room, but feels better for sleeping and fresh air, the chances are that Aconite will be the most appropriate remedy for the initial stage of this sore throat.

• Finally check with the **Keynotes** section at the back of the book that this is the remedy that matches your child's symptoms most closely. Remember that Aconite is a remedy that is most useful for the early symptoms of a sore throat, and that if your child moves on to a different stage of a cold, she may need a change of remedy that accommodates this shift. Also bear in mind that you can combine information from different tables: for example, if your child has a head cold and a cough, you can combine the **Cold** and **Cough** tables to find the most appropriate remedy that covers your child's symptoms as a whole.

• It is unlikely that a homoeopathic remedy will abort a sore throat or cold, but if your selection is appropriate, it will take your child through the various stages quickly, and with the minimum amount of discomfort and complication.

For information on how to administer the appropriate remedy, see the section entitled *Giving homoeopathic remedies to children* in Chapter 2 since exactly the same principles apply.

Croup

TYPE	GENERAL INDICATIONS	WORSE FROM	BETTER FOR	REMEDY NAME
Early stage of croup with marked anxiety and restlessness	Child wakes from sleep with dry, hoarse coughing fit. Fearful to the point of being convinced that they will die. Croupy cough comes on after midnight. Croup may follow on from exposure to cold, dry wind.	At night. Being cold. Drinking cold water. Exposure to tobacco smoke	Open air. Perspiring	Aconite
Croupy cough that causes wakefulness before midnight	Child may be woken from sleep before midnight, with a loud, dry cough which causes a feeling of suffocation. Croup with a very harsh, rasping cough that resembles a saw being drawn through dry wood.	Lying down. Talking. Very cold drinks. Breathing in. Movement	Warm drinks	Spongia
Ringing, croupy cough that begins the minute the head touches the pillow	Tickling in larynx precedes violent coughing spasms. Attacks often set in after midnight, especially around 2 a.m. Coughing fits may be so severe that they end in vomiting and cold sweats.	Lying down. After midnight. Talking. Eating. Cold drinks	Being active. Open air	Drosera

TYPE	GENERAL INDICATIONS	WORSE FROM	BETTER FOR	REMEDY NAME
Croupy, barking cough with marked sensitivity to cold draughts	Symptoms may be much worse in the morning and evening. Chilly with a marked preference for warmth: much worse from exposure to cold. Relief obtained from warm drinks.	Cold air. Touch. Pressure. Breathing out (the opposite of Spongia)	Warmth. Damp atmosphere	Hepar sulph
Croup which is very distressing and suffocating as child is entering a deep sleep.	Wakes with croupy coughing and choking sensation. It may be difficult to swallow because of constricted feeling in the larynx. Reacts badly to any feeling of pressure or constriction around the neck, from clothing or bedcovers.	Waking from sleep. Touch or even, light pressure on throat. Empty swallowing. Mornings	Open air. Cold drinks. Movement	Lachesis
Croupy cough with rawness and hoarseness in larynx	Croupy cough brought on by lying down at night or exposure to change of temperature. Difficulty breathing from tightness in chest. Anxiety is relieved by reassurance. Croup which has passed the violent stage of recent onset, but keeps relapsing.	Moving from one temperature to another. Exposure to strong odours. Talking	Warmth. Sitting propped up. Touch	Phosphorus

TYPE	GENERAL INDICATIONS	WORSE FROM	BETTER FOR	REMEDY NAME
Brassy-sounding croup with mucus that is stringy and difficult to move	Impulse to cough results in gagging and breathlessness. Symptoms may be worse in the morning or after eating. Wakes with feeling of pressure and heaviness in the chest.	Eating. Drinking. Uncovering. Open air. Waking. Stooping	Warmth. Movement. Bringing up mucus	Kali bich

General advice

In addition to homoeopathic prescribing, the following measures may be helpful:

- Move your child to the bathroom, turn on the hot water taps and hot shower and keep the doors and windows closed. If you sit in the room with your child to reassure him, a steamy atmosphere will often help the symptoms of croup subside fairly quickly. Make sure you stay with your child to guard against any accidental burning, from contact with hot taps or hot water.
- Reassure your child as much as possible: the symptoms of croup can cause great anxiety and distress to both children and parents. Panic can make the symptoms worse.

When to seek medical advice
If any of the following occurs, seek professional advice:

- Any sign of blueness around the lips or drooling from the mouth, with breathing difficulties.
- If steam hasn't helped within twenty minutes.
- If your child is distressed or the condition is worsening.

Sore throats

TYPE	GENERAL INDICATIONS	WORSE FROM	BETTER FOR	REMEDY NAME
Sore throat brought on by exposure to cold, dry winds	Rapid onset of symptoms with extreme anxiety and restlessness. High temperature with burning head and cold body. Hypersensitivity to pain. Most appropriate for the initial stages of sore throats.	Extreme changes of temperature. Warm rooms. At night. Being chilled	Sleep. Open air	Aconite
Violent, rapid onset of symptoms with high fever	High temperature with very dry, red, hot skin: skin radiates heat. Delirious state. Symptoms develop rapidly with throbbing, pulsating pains which are aggravated by the least movement. Dryness of throat which feels on fire. Difficulty swallowing.	Stimulation. Jolting or jarring. Exposure to cold	Warmth. Resting	Belladonna

TYPE	GENERAL INDICATIONS	WORSE FROM	BETTER FOR	REMEDY NAME
Sore throats with swollen glands which feel better for warm drinks	General sensitivity to cold draughts of air with illness. Generally sensitive and irritable. Sticking pains in throat: pains may radiate to the ears. Tonsils may become enlarged and ulcerated.	Cold draughts. Cold food or drinks. Touch. Morning and evening	Warmth. Warm, wet weather. After eating	Hepar sulph
Left-sided sore throats which are better for eating	Sore throat may be left-sided, or begin on the right and move to the left. Pain in the throat is worse after sleep and for empty swallowing (saliva). External throat very sensitive to touch.	Sleep. Left side. Pressure on throat. Swallow-ing saliva. Heat	Swallowing food. Open air. Cold drinks	Lachesis
Sore throats with swollen glands, increased saliva	Saliva increased with sore throats and flabby enlarged-looking tongue. Breath and perspiration smell offensive. Metallic taste in the mouth. Drowsy by day, restless at night. Ulcerated tonsils.	Extremes of tempera-ture. Warmth of bed. At night. Eating	Resting. Moderate tempera-tures	Mercurius

TYPE	GENERAL INDICATIONS	WORSE FROM	BETTER FOR	REMEDY NAME
Sore throat with stiff neck and swollen glands	Pain radiates from the throat into the ears on swallowing. Right-sided pain. Tonsils may become chronically enlarged. The throat looks dark red, purple or bluish. Pain felt at the base of the tongue when it is protruded. Feels bruised all over with illness.	Cold. Touch. Hot drinks	Warmth.	Phytolacca
Very swollen, puffy interior to throat: pains are much worse from heat in any form	Throat looks swollen, rosy-red and glossy. Water-logged appearence of throat especially of the uvula. Pains are severe and stinging and feel soothed by cool drinks.	Heat in any form. Touch or pressure. Lying down	Cool drinks. Cool air. Movement	Apis

Please refer to laryngitis (on page 104) for general advice and indications for seeking professional help.

Laryngitis

TYPE	GENERAL INDICATIONS	WORSE FROM	BETTER FOR	REMEDY NAME
Laryngitis with burning and severe hoarseness with loss of voice	Burning sensations in throat are relieved temporarily by cool drinks. All symptoms may feel worse in the evening. Marked anxiety accompanies illness. Dry cough with throat symptoms and constant desire to clear the throat.	Cold air. Touch. Speaking. Excitement. Being alone	Cold drinks. Sound sleep. Reassurance	Phosphorus
Rapid onset of loss of voice after chill or exposure to cold, dry winds	Dry, croupy cough with laryngitits and intense thirst for cold drinks. Indicated in the early stage of illness where there is marked anxiety, restlessness and fear. Symptoms are more intense at night.	Warm rooms. Exposure to cold, dry winds. Night. Eating or drinking. Talking	Open air. Rest	Aconite

TYPE	GENERAL INDICATIONS	WORSE FROM	BETTER FOR	REMEDY NAME
Hoarseness which is made much worse for exposure to cold draughts	A barking cough and sore throat which extend to the ears with hoarseness. General irritability and hypersensitivity. Feels better generally for exposure to warmth.	Cold air. Morning. Uncovering	Warmth. After eating. Warm wraps to the head	Hepar sulph
Hoarseness with ropy, stringy and yellow mucus	Cough with hoarseness, with a frequent desire to cough up mucus that is difficult to dislodge. Troublesome irritation at the back of the tongue. Soreness of the throat may be relieved by drinking hot fluids.	After eating. Drinking. Uncovering. Cold weather. After sleep	Lying in a warm bed. Warmth. Movement	Kali bich
Loss of voice which follows emotional distress or sudden shock	Hoarseness may be accompanied by a troublesome feeling of constriction in the throat. This may be so severe that the sensation resembles a ball or lump rising into the gullet. There may be general feelings of tightness or tension.	Yawning. Cold. Strong smells	Warmth. Eating. Distraction	Ignatia

General advice

In addition to homoeopathic prescribing, the following advice may also be helpful:

- Withhold foods that are difficult to swallow, or acidic drinks such as orange juice that make the throat feel more painful.
- Avoid exposing your child to marked changes of temperature: try to keep room temperature as stable as possible.
- Make sure your child drinks as much as possible. Plain water is best, but if your child is not keen on drinking liquids which are lacking in flavour, try introducing non-acidic drinks, or even ice-lollies, to make taking liquids more attractive.
- Use a humidifier, or humidify the air yourself by placing bowls of water at strategic points, e.g. near radiators.

When to seek medical advice
If any of the following occur, seek professional advice:

- Severe pain and difficulty swallowing.
- Any sign of drooling from the mouth.
- Breathing difficulties.
- Severe throat in a child with a family history of rheumatic fever.

Colds

TYPE	GENERAL INDICATIONS	WORSE FROM	BETTER FOR	REMEDY NAME
Rapid onset of symptoms after exposure to cold winds (early stage)	Rapid onset of violent, feverish symptoms with anxiety and restlessness. Sensitivity to light and marked thirst. Violent headaches accompany a runny, watery nasal discharge. Colds can follow a fright or shock.	Warm rooms. At night. Talking	Open air	Aconite
Colds which begin with rapidly-developing high temperature (early stage)	Symptoms are of violent intensity and develop very quickly. Skin is hot, dry and bright red: so hot it seems to radiate heat. Marked irritability with feverishness and intolerance of light and noise. Rapid pulse.	Stimulation of any kind. Light. Noise. Movement	Sitting propped up in bed	Belladonna
Early stage with flushing of the face which is confined to separate circular patches	Flushing is not so intensely hot as that which requires Belladonna, and less restless than those who need Aconite. Well-defined, circular patches of heat on cheeks. Nose bleeds may accompany cold symptoms.	At night. Movement. Cold air	Resting	Ferrum phos

TYPE	GENERAL INDICATIONS	WORSE FROM	BETTER FOR	REMEDY NAME
Terrific chilliness with cold symptoms and desire for warmth	Chilliness with marked desire for warmth in general: warm drinks, hot water bottles, or central heating turned up full. Lots of anxiety and restlessness with symptoms which are much worse at night.	Cold. At night. Being alone	Warmth. Company. Rest. Open air (especially if there is a headache)	Arsenicum album
Marked irritability with cold symptoms and sensitivity to draughts of cold air	Irritable and bad-tempered with illness. Very physically and mentally over-sensitive. May be constipated since having a cold. Nose feels blocked indoors and runs when out of doors. Nasal passages become very blocked at night. Repeated and distressing bouts of sneezing.	Draughts of cold air. Disturbed sleep. After eating. Touch. After waking	Napping. As the day goes on. Resting. Warmth	Nux vomica
Head colds with a burning nasal discharge that makes the nostrils and upper lip sore	Eyes may be watery with cold symptoms, but tears feel bland, even though the eyes may look bloodshot. Nasal discharge is clear and acrid: frequent sneezing that feels better out of doors.	Warm rooms. Indoors. Evenings	Out of doors. Cool rooms	Allium cepa

TYPE	GENERAL INDICATIONS	WORSE FROM	BETTER FOR	REMEDY NAME
Colds with nasal discharge like egg white and lots of sneezing.	Nose alternates between running like a tap or being blocked up. Cold sores may appear on the lips during a cold: lips may be dry and cracked. Thirst may be marked.	Warm rooms. Exposure to sun. Sympathy. After sleep	Not eating. Open, cool air	Natrum mur
Colds with profuse watery, bland discharge from nose.	Eyes may water with colds and feel very irritated. Eyelids may look red and swollen and feel sensitive to light. Chilly with frequent sneezing.	Coughing. Light. Wind. Night. Lying down	During the day	Euphrasia

For adjunctive measures, see section following the **Influenza** table.

Influenza ('flu)

TYPE	GENERAL INDICATIONS	WORSE FROM	BETTER FOR	REMEDY NAME
Early stage of 'flu with high temperature and hot, flushed, dry skin	Sudden onset of 'flu symptoms with high temperature and rapid pulse. Very hot, dry radiating skin, with general irritability and restlessness. Throat may burn and feel very dry with resulting difficulty in swallowing. Symptoms develop and resolve abruptly: may be right-sided.	Movement. Bright light. Noise. At night	Dark rooms. Resting	Belladonna

TYPE	GENERAL INDICATIONS	WORSE FROM	BETTER FOR	REMEDY NAME
Initial onset of 'flu symptoms after exposure to dry, cold winds, or from shock	Tremendous restlessness and anxiety with general symptoms. Symptoms appear with rapidity and violence. Terrific sensitivity to pains. Alternately dry and hot, looking alternately pale and flushed.	At night. In the evening. Being touched	Fresh air	Aconite
'Flu with terrible aching and restlessness	Everything feels achey: bones, head, eyes and skin. Although feverish there is little sweat, but a strong thirst. Yawns and feels sleepy most of the time. Aching is preceded by sneezing and redness of the eyes. Very chilly: wants to be kept covered.	Open air. Uncovering	Indoors. Distraction	Eupatorium perfoliatum
Slow-developing symptoms after exposure to extremes of temperature	Fever is slow to develop: child complains of feeling generally unwell for a few days before symptoms appear. Muscle aches and headache which are made much worse by motion. Dry mouth and skin with thirst for cold drinks. Grumpy with illness.	Motion. Warm rooms. Cold drinks. Sympathy	Cool rooms. Open air. Sweating	Bryonia

TYPE	GENERAL INDICATIONS	WORSE FROM	BETTER FOR	REMEDY NAME
'Flu with aching, shivering and terrific weariness.	Eyelids look and feel heavy and droopy: the child generally looks and feels extremely lethargic. Very chilly and wants to stay warm. Lack of thirst although feverish. Easily exhausted by the least movement. Slow-developing symptoms like Bryonia.	Cold draughts. Hot rooms. Direct sunlight	Sweating. Passing water	Gelsemium
Marked chilliness, restlessness and anxiety with 'flu symptoms	Terrible anxiety with the onset of symptoms that gets much worse at night. Responds well to warmth in general, but feels better for fresh air if there is an accompanying headache. Burning pains: nostrils red and sore from nasal discharge. Seems weaker and more distressed than the severity of the illness warrants.	Cold. At night	Sips of warm drinks. Warmth. Company	Arsenicum album

TYPE	GENERAL INDICATIONS	WORSE FROM	BETTER FOR	REMEDY NAME
'Flu symptoms with constant tossing and turning at night	Generalised aching and stiffness with 'flu symptoms. Constant movement relieves: keeping still makes the child feel worse. Fever and aching are worse at night when in bed. There may be alternating feverishness and chilliness.	At night. Warmth of bed. Keeping still. Over-exertion	Warm bathing. Gentle movement. Wrapping up warmly	Rhus tox

General advice

In addition to homoeopathic prescribing, the following advice may be useful:

- Make sure your child is not exposed to extreme changes of temperature: avoid going outside at all if it is cold or windy, and avoid bathing your child if he or she is feverish.
- Encourage as much rest or sleep as possible.
- Provided your child is kept warm and not chilled, you can try to see if fresh air makes him or her more comfortable.
- Use a humidifier as suggested in the previous section.
- Avoid mucus-forming foods as much as possible such as cow's milk and dairy products in general.
- Gently clear the nostrils of a very small child or baby before they feed by using a tissue, making sure you don't push the mucus inwards.
- Tilt the head end of your infant's mattress by putting one or two pillows underneath it (not directly under an

infant's head). This encourages mucus to drain downwards from the nose. Alternatively, put some books under the legs of the head end of the cot/bed, to elevate it, achieving the same purpose.

- Keep the diet as light as possible, avoiding any foods that are difficult to digest. Make sure that the liquid content is high by encouraging your child to drink as much water as possible. This is very important if your child has a raised temperature.
- Avoid using aspirin since it may be implicated in the development of Reye's Syndrome. This is a serious illness which is characterised by symptoms of high temperature, vomiting and liver and kidney problems.

When to seek medical advice
If any of the following occur, seek professional advice:

- Raised temperature, accompanied by lethargy, stiff neck, irritability or changed breathing pattern.
- Stubborn raised temperature that does not respond to homoeopathic or naturopathic measures.
- Any signs of wheezing.
- If vomiting occurs during the course of the illness.
- If your child is subject to repeated bouts of cold symptoms, you need to consult a homoeopathic practitioner in order to deal with your child's predisposition to the problem. For an explanation of why this is necessary, see Chapter 7, **Chronic and Long-Term Problems in Children,** on page 135.

Coughs

TYPE	GENERAL INDICATIONS	WORSE FROM	BETTER FOR	REMEDY NAME
Dry, tickly cough that is worse at night and for lying down in bed	Chilliness, anxiety and restlessness with wheezy cough that feels better for warmth. Symptoms are worse after midnight until 2 a.m. Feels better for sips of warm drinks although there are burning sensations with the cough.	At night. Cold. Lying down. Eating or drinking. Exertion	Warmth. Sitting up. Being indoors. Company	Arsenicum album
Dry, tickly, irritating cough with gagging or vomiting that is much worse for moving around	Tickly cough which may be set off or made worse by entering a warm room. Cough may be so distressing that child holds on to, or presses against, chest for relief. Coughing fits may be temporarily relieved by cold drinks. Very irritable and bad-tempered since cough set in: wants to be left undisturbed.	Warm surroundings. Being wrapped up. Slightest movement. Being disturbed	Lying still. Firm pressure. Cool rooms and cool drinks	Bryonia

TYPE	GENERAL INDICATIONS	WORSE FROM	BETTER FOR	REMEDY NAME
Harsh, croupy-sounding cough that follows exposure to cold, dry winds	Very restless and anxious with cough that sounds barking and choking. Most useful in the early stage of a croupy cough, especially if the onset has been sudden. Goes to bed seeming fine, but wakes in the first half of the night very distressed and coughing.	Extreme temperatures. At night. Warm rooms. Lying down. Attempting to talk	Open air. Being able to sleep	Aconite
Loud, rattly cough with great difficulty in bringing up phlegm	Useful in the later stages of a cough. There may be drowsiness, lethargy and irritability with illness. Coughing spasms may be especially severe towards 4 a.m. Chilly, but doesn't like to be kept in a warm room. Needs to sit up when coughing.	Stuffy rooms. Warmth. Towards morning. Getting angry. Eating. Damp conditions. Lying down	Cool air. Sitting up. Bringing up phlegm	Antimonium tart
Choking, suffocating coughing bouts that come on as soon as the head touches the pillow	Hoarseness and suffocative spasms which come on when eating, talking or drinking cold drinks. Although chilly, coughing is accompanied by profuse sweating, especially at night. May vomit with cough.	Lying down. At 2 a.m. Cold drinks. Eating. Laughing	Open air. Being active	Drosera

TYPE	GENERAL INDICATIONS	WORSE FROM	BETTER FOR	REMEDY NAME
Bouts of coughing with vomiting and retching	Paleness may be marked with illness, or during coughing bouts; the face may become flushed and bright red. Cough may be dry and tickling, or wheezy and rattling. Awful nausea with cough. Lots of bad temper and screaming accompanies feeling ill. Symptoms develop quickly, unlike Antimonium tart.	Eating. Cold weather. Humid weather. Being touched	Open air. Firm pressure. Sitting up	Ipecac
Cough which is dry, hard and wheezy, and made worse by moving from warm room to cold air	Lots of anxiety with coughing and tightness in the chest. Craving for ice-cold drinks. Exhausted from coughing spasms and relieved by being warm in bed. Burning pains in chest. Mucus discharges are yellowy-green in colour, and may contain streaks of blood. Feels better for attention and reassurance.	Lying on the left side. Strong smells. Changing from one temperature to another. Evenings	Warmth. Sympathy. Reassurance. Cold drinks	Phosphorus

TYPE	GENERAL INDICATIONS	WORSE FROM	BETTER FOR	REMEDY NAME
Terrific sensitivity to cold air with tickly cough and hoarseness	Child may pull blanket over his or her head to avoid breathing in cold air which triggers their coughing spasms. Very sensitive throat-pit to touch, with lots of irritation in the larynx. Hacking, barking cough prevents sleep.	Cold air. Movement. At night. Touching the external throat	Warm air. Covering mouth with a scarf	Rumex crispus.
Cough which is accompan-ied by productive green mucus which builds up overnight	Symptoms are made generally worse by being in stuffy rooms, and improved by gentle movement in the fresh air. Also worse for lying down and resting. Cough will be alternately dry during the day and loose overnight and on waking. Clingy and weepy during illness, requiring a lot of attention and sympathy.	Warm rooms. Stuffy atmo-spheres. Warm weather. Lying flat	Cool, fresh air. Gentle motion. Sympathy and attention	Pulsatilla

TYPE	GENERAL INDICATIONS	WORSE FROM	BETTER FOR	REMEDY NAME
Barking, dry, hollow cough which may be brought on by over-excitement	Breathing may be difficult because of constant, irritating coughing fits. Bruised and sore feelings in the chest. Cough is especially severe on waking from sleep, causing anxiety and distress. Eating sweets can also lead to a coughing bout.	Sleep. Exercise. Talking. Tight clothes	Warmth. Eating and drinking	Spongia tosta
Persistent, lingering coughs that do not clear up after indicated remedy has been given	Cough follows a chill or exposure to dampness in winter. Irritating, slow-developing cough with thick, lumpy, yellow mucus. Exhaustion and general weariness with cough	Being chilled. Uncovering head or feet. First thing in the morning	Warm or hot drinks. Wrapping up snuggly: especially involving the head. Being warm in bed	Silica

General advice

In addition to homoeopathic prescribing, the following measures may be useful:

• Avoid mucus-forming products such as cow's milk. Take special care to avoid giving a milky drink at night: this can encourage a build-up of mucus as the night progresses.

• Use a humidifier at all times or place bowls of water near radiators.

- Encourage your child to drink as much as possible to encourage loosening of mucus.
- Try to keep as calm as possible and reassure your child during a coughing fit, especially if coughing is accompanied by vomiting which can cause great distress: panicking makes breathing much more difficult.
- Encourage a baby to bring up mucus by letting her lie face-down over your knees with her bottom slightly more raised than her chest. Gently pat her back to help expel mucus. Infants and older children can be encouraged to lean slightly forwards during a coughing spasm.
- Avoid exposing your child to extreme changes of temperature.
- Encourage your child to eat little and often if vomiting accompanies the cough, trying to time the snacks at the end of a coughing bout.
- Encourage as much sleep and rest as possible.

When to seek medical advice
If any of the following occur seek professional help:

- Distressed, irregular, wheezy or laboured breathing.
- Chest pain.
- Accelerated breathing
- Persistent vomiting with coughing bouts in babies immediately after feeding.
- Fever in babies which is accompanied by rapid breathing, lethargy and paleness.
- Extreme drowsiness or confusion.
- Suspicion that a foreign body may have been inhaled.
- Persistent coughing that has not responded to reasonable

self-help measures, especially if it is accompanied by a
general malaise and decline in well-being.

Earache

TYPE	GENERAL INDICATIONS	WORSE FROM	BETTER FOR	REMEDY NAME
Ear pain which sets in after exposure to dry, cold winds	Symptoms are sudden in onset and violent in nature. External ear is painful and hot. There may be general hypersensitivity to pain, noise and music. Temperature is high with profound restlessness and anxiety.	Cold winds. Warm rooms. In the evening and at night. Lying on the painful side	Open, fresh air. After perspiring	Aconite
Earache with high temperature and very red, flushed, hot face	Sudden, violent onset of symptoms. Ear in general looks bright red and inflamed. Right side may be more affected than the left and throbbing pains shoot to the throat. Soreness of throat, and glandular swelling. Extreme irritability and agitation with illness. Indicated in the early stages	Movement and jarring. Noise. Stimulation. Cold air. At night	Warm applications. Resting semi-propped-up in bed	Belladonna

TYPE	GENERAL INDICATIONS	WORSE FROM	BETTER FOR	REMEDY NAME
Earache with screaming and extreme irritability	Pain causes such distress that child cannot be pacified: throws toys that are offered to the floor in temper and frustration. Earache accompanies teething and is worse for exposure to cold air. One cheek may look hot and bright red, while the other may be pale and cool.	Light. Noise. Touch. Heat. Warm rooms. Cold winds	Being rocked or carried. Being driven in a car	Chamomilla
Early stage of earache with symptoms that are milder than those which require Aconite or Belladonna	Flushed or pale with pain, or may alternate between the two. Drawing sensations in the ear with possible itching. Indicated for the early stage of earache where pus has not yet formed. Pain may be restricted to the left side.	Open air. Exertion. Noise	Gentle motion	Ferrum phos
Earache with terrific sensitivity to cold draughts	Lots of irritability and bad temper with pains. The minute a limb is exposed to cold air, child demands to be covered. Aversion to being touched when sick and in pain. Discharge is thick, yellow and offensive-smelling, with sticking, sharp pains in throat and ears.	Cold winds and draughts. Lying on the painful side. At night. Fresh air	Warm wraps to the head. Being warm in bed. Heat in general	Hepar sulph

TYPE	GENERAL INDICATIONS	WORSE FROM	BETTER FOR	REMEDY NAME
Earache with offensive discharge and sore throat and swollen glands	Discharge from the ear is offensive-smelling, as well as the breath. Colour of discharge is yellow or green. Increased saliva: child dampens the pillow through drooling overnight. Sweat is also increased.	At night. Warmth of bed. Extremes of temperature. Stooping. Touch and pressure	Moderate temperatures. During the day. At rest	Mercurius
Later, established stage of ear infection with weepiness	Although chilly with illness, child feels worse for stuffy rooms and craves cool, fresh air. Discharge is thick and creamy or yellowy-green. Earache follows on from getting chilled or wet. Easily comforted during illness by sympathy and attention.	Night. In bed. Humidity. Warm food or drinks	Fresh, open air. Gentle motion. Cool food. Cool applications. Sympathy	Pulsatilla

General advice

The following measures may be helpful in addition to homoeopathic prescribing:

- Make sure your child drinks as much fluid as possible.
- Avoid exposure to cold winds.
- Use warm applications such as a hot water bottle wrapped in a towel to hold against the ear, or a cool pack

wrapped in fabric, depending on which your child feels is more soothing. Always make sure that the hot water bottle is securely wrapped up and is not in danger of coming in direct contact with your infant's skin.

- Look out for tell-tale signs of ear problems in a baby or infant such as crying, rubbing or pulling on the ear.
- Do not attempt to clean out the ear yourself: if you suspect ear problems take your child to be examined by your GP or homoeopathic practitioner.
- Avoid contact with water while the ear is recovering.
- If your child suffers from repeated ear infections it is advisable to seek the help and advice of a homoeopathic practitioner.

When to seek medical advice
If any of the following occur, seek professional advice:

- Severe pain, especially if accompanied by swelling, redness, sensitivity or pain behind the ear.
- If self-help measures are not helping within twenty-four hours.
- Depressed or swollen fontanelle (the soft spot at the crown of the head) in babies.
- Discharge from the ear which is bloody, clear or pussy.
- If you suspect that a foreign body may have found its way into your child's ear, do not attempt to remove it yourself but take him or her for professional help. There is always the danger that you may inadvertently push the object more deeply into the ear.
- If you are concerned about the general severity of any symptoms.

Styes

TYPE	GENERAL INDICATIONS	WORSE FROM	BETTER FOR	REMEDY NAME
Styes that are very rosy, swollen, glossy-looking with stinging pains	Tears sting and burn. Pain is relieved by cold bathing and made much worse by heat and warmth.	Heat. Warm bathing of the affected area. Touch or pressure. At night. After sleep	Cool air. Cool bathing. Movement	Apis
Rapidly developing styes where the eye looks red and dry	Marked sensitivity to light and pupils may be dilated. Strong irritability and bad temper with eye symptoms. Area around the eye feels very swollen, pounding and throbbing.	Light. Jarring. Lying on the affected side	Rest. Darkened rooms	Belladonna
Styes which are made worse by warm applications	Recurring styes on the lower lid. Discharges are greeny-yellow. Pain is made easier by cold compresses held against the affected area. Lids stick together after sleep and feel very itchy. Constant feeling of wanting to rub the lids for relief.	Heat. Resting. Stuffy rooms. Warm applications	Cool, fresh air. Cool applica-tions. Gentle exercise out of doors	Pulsatilla

TYPE	GENERAL INDICATIONS	WORSE FROM	BETTER FOR	REMEDY NAME
Styes which are acutely sensitive to cold air	Exposure to cold winds causes great distress and irritability. Stye looks very swollen and may exude a yellowish, thick discharge. Feels much better for general and local heat. Pains are sharp and sticking.	Cold draughts. Light touch. Pressure	Warmth	Hepar sulph
Styes which feel hot and are much worse for bathing	Lids burn and itch and look very red around the edges. Eyes water a lot and lids may stick together after sleep. Reacts very badly to heat in any form.	Warmth. Severe cold. Bathing	Moderate temperatures. Cool air. Scratching	Sulphur

General advice

In addition to homoeopathic prescribing, the following advice may be helpful:

- Try to discourage your child from rubbing or scratching her eyes where possible; clipping finger nails quite short can be helpful.
- Consider the amount of sugar in your child's diet: if it is high, reduce it as much as possible. It has been suggested that refined sugar, which can be found in cakes, biscuits, ice-cream and carbonated drinks, can contribute to an environment which encourages the growth of bacteria. If

your child has a high sugar intake, and suffers from recurrent styes, his diet may be part of the problem.
- If styes are recurring at regular intervals, your child could benefit from long-term homoeopathic help from a professional practitioner.

Vomiting and diarrhoea

TYPE	GENERAL INDICATIONS	WORSE FROM	BETTER FOR	REMEDY NAME
Vomiting and diarrhoea which follow eating spoiled fruit	Classic food poisoning picture where vomiting and diarrhoea occur simultaneously. Very chilly, sweaty, anxious, restless or completely prostrate. Responds very well to warmth in general, even though pains may feel burning. Very fearful and panicky with illness.	Cold in any form. At night. Exertion. Taking food or cold drinks. Least touch	Warmth. Sips of warm drinks (cold drinks are vomited straight back). Bed rest	Arsenicum album
Violent vomiting and diarrhoea with marked thirst for cold water	Exhausting bouts of diarrhoea and vomiting which occur alternately leading to pallor, cold sweat and chilliness. May look on the verge of collapse. Vomiting and diarrhoea are forcible. After vomiting constant thirst for ice-cold water; aversion to warm drinks.	Moving. Touch. Warmth. At night	Resting. Lying down. Coolness	Veratrum album

TYPE	GENERAL INDICATIONS	WORSE FROM	BETTER FOR	REMEDY NAME
Diarrhoea and vomiting with terrible nausea that is much worse for slightest movement	Awful nausea which neither vomiting nor diarrhoea relieve, even temporarily. Very sensitive to the least movement which intensifies the nausea. Onset of symptoms is rapid with marked exhaustion. Constant desire to open bowels.	Cold. Extreme heat. Movement. Being disturbed	Resting. Closing eyes	Ipecac
Distressing nausea with difficulty in vomiting	Picture of 'reverse peristalsis' where there are difficulties in raising vomit or in emptying bowels: discharges refuse to be fully expelled. Problems may come on after over-eating. Pains are cramping and are relieved by passing a stool.	Cold in general. Being woken from sleep. Tight clothes. After eating	Being left undisturbed to nap. Warmth. Passing wind. Hot drinks	Nux vomica
Empty retching with gushing, involuntary diarrhoea	Watery, frothy diarrhoea that is preceded by awful nausea: gagging with diarrhoea. Lots of gurgling in abdomen and bowels with colicky pains. Symptoms are often worse in the morning.	Touch. Motion. Morning (especially early morning). Open air	Rubbing. Lying on abdomen. External heat	Podophyllum

TYPE	GENERAL INDICATIONS	WORSE FROM	BETTER FOR	REMEDY NAME
Vomiting with violent retching and watery stools that smell like rotten eggs	Very distressed and irritable with illness. Screams and cannot be consoled. Effort of retching leads to cold sweat and exhaustion. Colicky pains make child double up and kick and scream. Bright red in the face from screaming outbursts. Diarrhoea accompanies teething pains.	Draughts of cold air. In the first part of the night	Local heat to the abdomen. Being rocked, carried, or driven in a car	Chamomilla
Colicky pains with vomiting and diarrhoea, with vast accumulation of wind	Very sensitive on mental and physical levels: pains seem intolerable. Very restless with pains, keeping still makes things worse. When pains build, nausea and vomiting begin. Retching continues until stomach has been completely emptied. Diarrhoea has a yellowish tinge.	Exposure to cold. Eating fruit. Keeping still. Afternoons	Hard pressure. Lying on abdomen. Bending double. Heat locally applied. Passing wind	Colocythis

TYPE	GENERAL INDICATIONS	WORSE FROM	BETTER FOR	REMEDY NAME
Stomach upsets from eating overly-rich, greasy or fatty foods	Symptoms may set in after too rich a diet or getting severely chilled and damp. Nausea and vomiting is accompanied by terrible chills, but warm rooms make child feel worse. Burning sensations in stomach are aggravated by warm foods, and temporarily relieved by cold. Nocturnal diarrhoea with burning sensations in bowel. Very weepy and clingy when ill.	Stuffy rooms. At night. Resting. Warm food and drinks. Getting chilled	Fresh air. Gentle movement. Sympathy and attention. Cold foods and drinks	Pulsatilla

General advice

In addition to homoeopathic prescribing, the following advice may be helpful:

• Do not push unwanted food on your child when vomiting and/or diarrhoea are present. Where these two conditions occur, the digestive tract is often attempting to deal with an infection by expelling the content of the stomach and bowel. Eating can make this process more protracted and uncomfortable.

However, it is essential to ensure that dehydration does not occur by encouraging your child to drink as much as possible. The best fluid is water: avoid giving orange juice or milk which are likely to irritate the digestive tract further. When diarrhoea and vomiting occur together, dehydration can happen quite rapidly, especially in a very small child or baby. For a list of signs of dehydration see section on **Colic** in Chapter 5.

- Reassure and comfort your child as much as possible during and after vomiting: it can be an extremely frightening and distressing experience which can be made worse by panic.
- Sponging your child's face after being sick may feel comforting.

When to seek medical advice
If any of the following occur, seek professional advice:

- Signs of dehydration.
- Constant vomiting.
- If your child is in distress and inconsolable, or if you are concerned about the severity of the symptoms.
- Signs of blood in vomit or stools, or dark-coloured vomit.
- Vomiting or nausea which follows a fall on the head.
- Severe pain in the abdomen, especially if it is accompanied by tenderness, vomiting, diarrhoea and raised temperature.

Constipation

TYPE	GENERAL INDICATIONS	WORSE FROM	BETTER FOR	REMEDY NAME
Slow-developing symptoms with marked thirst	Very grumpy and irritable with constipation: wants to be left alone. Very sensitive to heat and motion: feels worse for both. Complains of dry mouth and throat and wants lots of cold drinks. Headache with constipation that is made worse by stooping. Stools are large, hard and dry.	Warmth. Movement. Sympathy. Bending forwards	Keeping still. Being left undisturbed. Cool in general. Darkened rooms	Bryonia
Constipation with general sluggishness and no urge to pass a stool	Stools are soft, small, knotted or dry. Whatever the nature of the stool, it is very difficult to pass. The rectum may be inflamed, sore and sensitive. Bleeding may occur from rawness. Foods that aggravate the condition include dry, starchy ingredients such as potatoes.	Sitting still. Eating rich or starchy foods	Warmth Warm foods or drinks. Cool bathing	Alumina

TYPE	GENERAL INDICATIONS	WORSE FROM	BETTER FOR	REMEDY NAME
Constipation with irritability and sensitivity to cold.	Headache, nausea, and constipation following over-indulgence in rich foods or a course of drugs. Syndrome of 'bashful stool' (stool keeps moving back in again) and incomplete bowel movements after straining. Constant urging and desire to pass a stool. Mental and physical over-sensitivity with constipation: very irritable.	Being cold. Fussing. Lack of, or interrupted, sleep. Noise	Undis-turbed sleep. Resting. Warmth	Nux vomica
Constipation from change in routine such as being away from home	Lots of rumbling, gurgling and wind which passes upwards and downwards with constipation. Very sensitive to pressure around the waist; wants to have clothing loosened. No desire to pass a stool for days, followed by days of constant urging.	Pressure. Feeling overheated. Cold food or drinks. Travel	Loosening clothing. Warm drinks. Being occupied and distracted. Open air	Lycopodium

General advice

The following measures will be helpful in addition to homoeopathic prescribing:

- Check that your child's diet includes the necessary amount of fibre from fresh fruit and vegetables: often re-introducing these foods will rectify the problem.
- Ensure that your child is drinking enough water as well as other drinks such as fresh (ideally unsweetened) fruit juice. Increasing fluid intake can make stools easier to pass.
- Avoid foods that have been cooked in aluminium containers, or drinks that use aluminium in their production, such as tea bags.
- Avoid, or use very sparingly, foods that take a long time to digest such as eggs, cheese, red meat, or other ingredients that are high in fat, if your child shows tendencies to constipation. Concentrate instead on foods that pass more quickly through the digestive tract such as fruit, vegetables and lighter forms of protein such as fish or poultry.
- Try to rectify the problem through dietary measures rather than resorting to laxatives. Although they produce results initially, they can lead to eventual aggravation of constipation by making the bowel increasingly more lax, and increasingly unable to work efficiently on its own.
- If your child's anus looks sore or inflamed after straining to pass a stool, apply Calendula ointment to the general area.
- The remedies suggested in the table above are only recommended for short-term use if your child has a brief bout of constipation. If this is beginning to be a regular,

or long-term problem, you need to seek professional
advice from a homoeopathic practitioner.

When to seek medical advice
If any of the following occur, seek professional sdvice:

- Signs of bleeding during, or after, passing a stool.
- Stools which are different in colour to normal, or which
  look very pale or very dark.
- Stubborn constipation which refuses to respond to self-
  help measures.
- Pain or distress on passing a stool.
- Alternation between diarrhoea and constipation.

CHAPTER 7

CHRONIC AND LONG-TERM PROBLEMS IN CHILDREN

A ll of the conditions described so far in this book will lend themselves to self-help measures, provided complications do not set in. This is because they are problems which fall into a disease category which is called acute. In other words, they are self-limiting illnesses which have a predictable life span which the body has the resources to resolve and deal with by itself. Within this context, the appropriate homoeopathic remedy is acting as a catalyst or booster, supporting and speeding up the healing processes which would happen naturally given enough time and support through good nursing.

However, there is another form of illness which is categorised as chronic. This does not refer to the severity or strength of a disease, but refers instead to a particular pattern or course of recurrent illness. For example, hay fever, eczema, psoriasis or asthma are illnesses which share common features of a chronic problem. These include:

- Repeated flare-ups or episodes of illness which continue over a long period of time.
- These episodes often remain static with regard to severity, or get progressively worse. Even though there are periods of remission, the body has difficulties resolving the

situation, however much time and opportunity it is given
to recover.

- Although some chronic problems can be resolved in time,
such as juvenile asthma which improves once a child has
passed through the teenage years, the general pattern of
chronic illness is that of repeated flare-ups which go into
abeyance for a while, but always tend to return.

Why chronic problems should not be treated by home prescribing

Homoeopathic treatment is eminently suitable for
treating chronic illness, provided treatment is
administered by a trained practitioner. The reasons for this
are straightforward and relate to the nature of the progression
of chronic disease.

Because a homoeopath works by searching for the
appropriately-chosen remedy that will stimulate the self-
healing capacity of the body as a whole, rather than
randomly prescribing more than one remedy for different
symptoms, case-analysis can be a complex and painstaking
business requiring years of training, skill and experience.
Although it is possible for a beginner to select an appropriate
homoeopathic remedy for an acute attack of asthma or hay
fever if the symptoms are well-defined, this will usually only
provide temporary help and is unlikely to deal with the
sufferer's predisposition to the problem.

For the latter to take place, it is necessary for a
professional homoeopath to spend an extended time with a
patient gathering a wide range of information regarding the

development of the current condition, a very detailed account of the symptoms, details of medical and family history, and as clear an impression as possible of the emotional make-up of that individual. For this process to take place, it is important that the homoeopath be as objective as possible. This is the main reason why many homoeopaths, in common with conventional doctors, will not treat members of their own family or close friends for a chronic condition.

Once an appropriate homoeopathic remedy has been selected and given for a chronic condition, assessing the progress of the case from this point can be a delicate and complex business. This is especially true where there are a number of related conditions as in the case of a child who suffers from eczema, asthma and hay fever. In this situation, very careful case management is needed to steer the patient towards an improved state of health. The practitioner needs to be prepared for any complications that may arise during treatment, and must constantly use his or her judgement to assess how the patient is progressing. Case-management of skin disorders can be especially delicate, and home-prescribing is emphatically discouraged for such conditions, since homoeopaths view a persistent skin eruption as an indication of a deeper, underlying, inherited disorder which needs to be dealt with before the whole person can enjoy an improved state of health.

This does not suggest that parents should not be empowered in taking an active role in improving the health of their children, or that they cannot contribute an essential amount of vital information and support if their child is being treated by a homoeopath. However, it is important to recognise both the value and the limitations of self-help prescribing, so that disappointing and discouraging results are avoided in situations where professional help is necessary to achieve a favourable outcome.

If your child is suffering from any of the conditions listed below, you should consult a homoeopathic practitioner rather than attempting to deal with it yourself. These include:

Asthma	*Eczema*
Anxiety	*Glue ear*
Bedwetting	*Hay fever*
Bronchitis	*Hyperactivity*
Colds which keep occurring	*Insomnia*
Constipation which is	*Psoriasis*
persistent	*Shyness or loss of confidence*
Eating disorders	*Warts*

CHAPTER 8

PRACTICAL INFORMATION: YOUR QUESTIONS ANSWERED

Where can I obtain homoeopathic medicines?

It is becoming increasingly easy to buy homoeopathic medicines since there are growing numbers of outlets emerging which sell these products in order to meet customer demand. Many pharmacies and high street chemists, including large chain stores such as Boots, will have a basic stock of homoeopathic remedies, while health food shops will often provide a reasonable choice.

An even more satisfactory source, with regard to availability and choice of different potencies, is provided by the number of homoeopathic pharmacies which manufacture and sell remedies. These have the added advantage of employing trained staff who can often answer basic questions relating to elementary homoeopathic prescribing, or who know where to refer you for further help and advice. These are also the best outlets to approach if you want to obtain a homoeopathic first-aid kit: they often have a selection of their own, or will be happy to put together one of your own choice. If you do not have a local homoeopathic pharmacy (see the **Useful Addresses** section), you can usually place orders in writing, or by telephone.

You can obtain homoeopathic medicines in the form of small or large tablets, granules, powders, pilules or in liquids. Creams, ointments, lotions and tinctures are also available for external use.

What does the word 'potency' refer to?

You will find that the homoeopathic medicines available to you in pharmacies and health shops usually come in a 6c potency, and sometimes in a 30c. The letter 'c' refers to the method of dilution that has been used (in this case the centesimal scale of dilution). This means that the original substance has been made into a liquid and diluted in an alcohol solution. One drop of this solution is added to ninety-nine drops of distilled water or alcohol and shaken or 'succussed' to render the first potency or 1c. This process is repeated at each stage, taking one drop of the last potency and adding it to ninety-nine drops of dilutant. Non-soluble substances such as metals or minerals go through a grinding process called 'trituration' in order to make them soluble.

You can also come across medicines that have a 'd', or 'x' after the number which means these have been diluted according to the decimal scale. This involves the same basic process that has been outlined above, but in this case the proportions used are one drop of dilutant to nine drops of alcohol or distilled water. When buying homoeopathic medicines, you may find that the 'c' is often omitted from the centesinal potencies. As a result, a centesinal potency of Arnica may be labelled 'Arnica 6' or 'Arnica 30'. However, decimal potencies will always have a 'd' or 'x' on the label.

Putting together a homoeopathic first-aid kit

Putting together a first-aid kit with children in mind is slightly different to selecting remedies for a more general kit. While homoeopathic medicines are not condition-specific (most medicines can be used for a wide range of differing conditions), there are certain medicines that have particular associations with the symptoms of childhood illness, such as Chamomilla.

It is very difficult to be absolutely specific about the optimum number of medicines included in a first-aid kit, since what is appropriate will vary according to individual needs. However, the following list will provide a sound basis for a children's starter kit, since it includes a basic range of the most frequently indicated homoeopathic remedies.

Aconite	*Gelsemium*
Arnica	*Hepar sulph*
Arsenicum album	*Nux vomica*
Belladonna	*Phosphorus*
Bryonia	*Pulsatilla*
Ferrum phos	*Rhus tox*

Once you have this basic range of remedies, the following would be useful additions to consider:

Apis	*Ledum*
Carbo veg	*Lycopodium*
Chamomilla	*Mercurius*
Drosera	*Lachesis*
Hypericum	*Ruta*

Ipecac	*Spongia*
Calc carb	*Sulphur*

Bear in mind that you can select medicines for your kit according to your individual requirements. For example, the remedies listed above are the most general suggestions for those which would be useful for any child from the toddler stage. However, if you have a baby you are intending to prescribe for, it would be helpful to include the following in your basic selection:

Borax	*Dioscorea*
Calc phos	*Kali mur*
Chamomilla	*Mag phos*
Colocynthis	*Kreosotum*

In addition, the following creams and tinctures are useful additions to a basic first-aid kit:

Calendula or Hypercal tincture or lotion: to be used diluted on cuts, bites, and grazes.
Calendula ointment or cream: should be used after bathing the affected area with diluted Calendula tincture to inhibit infection and to speed up the healing process.
Urtica urens lotion or tincture: to be diluted and applied to minor burns and scalds (no larger in diameter than a 2p piece).

These are general suggestions that can be added to, or changed according to your own needs. Although there are many other 'basic' homoeopathic medicines which are all useful, the lists given above will give you a good, sound basis for a practical kit which will cover most eventualities included in this book.

How do I know which potency to buy?

As before, this is a very difficult question to answer, since different situations require different potencies of the appropriate remedy. For a basic explanation of homoeopathic remedies and their potencies, please see the section entitled *What does the word 'potency' refer to?* earlier in this chapter. It is generally most practical when first buying your remedies to opt for a 6c potency, and to supplement these with the same medicines in a 12c or 30c as you gain more experience and enthusiasm for home prescribing. Don't worry unduly about selecting the optimum potency in the early days: provided you have selected the most appropriate remedy for your child, you can use whichever potency you have to hand. However, always bear in mind that a 6c potency will require more frequent repetition than a higher one.

When prescribing for your child always remember that conditions often develop more rapidly and violently in children, and that the remedy you have selected may need to be repeated more frequently in order to maintain an improvement. If the remedy seems to be giving only short-lived or partial relief in a 6c potency, consider moving on to the same remedy in a 12c or 30c. As always, avoid repeating the remedy while an improvement is holding; only use it again if there are signs of a relapse. If you are at all concerned about your child's condition, get professional advice.

Is there any risk of homoeopathic remedies producing side effects?

Because homoeopathic remedies stimulate the self-healing capacity of the body by boosting vital energy, side effects resulting from a toxic build-up in the body are unlikely to happen. However, it is wise to be aware that over-stimulation, through too frequent a repetition of a homoeopathic medicine, is something to be avoided. It is for this reason that you should always stop giving a remedy if you have observed a reaction. Any improvement in symptoms is a sign that your child's body has been stimulated into a curative response and that it can cope well under its own steam until a relapse occurs. If the latter happens, you can repeat the remedy until you see another improvement. Once this happens, always watch and wait rather than repeating the remedy. If a remedy has been very helpful but seems to have stopped being useful, take a closer look at the current presenting symptoms and see if another remedy is better indicated. If the symptoms have not changed, consider using a higher potency of the original remedy.

The main problem with too frequent administration of a homoeopathic remedy is that the original symptoms for which the remedy was given might briefly get more intense. If this happens, all that needs to be done is to stop giving the remedy, and, within a short space of time, things should return to where they were before the aggravation set in. On the other hand, if you give your child an inappropriately chosen remedy for a relatively short period of time (for instance, two or three doses over the same number of hours) the worst that is likely to happen is the disappointment of seeing no improvement in the symptoms. In this situation no

harm has been done; just return to the remedy table and take
a closer look at your child's symptoms to see if a closer match
can be obtained.

What if my child is already taking orthodox drugs, such as antibiotics?

Competently prescribed homoeopathic remedies can be
immensely useful in helping your child fight both
bacterial and viral infections. The results that are obtained
will depend very much on the skill and experience of the
prescriber, but appropriate use of homoeopathic medicines as
the first resort, often means that antibiotics can be reserved
for major infections that refuse to yield to more holistic
measures.

Although it is much more straightforward to prescribe
homoeopathically for a child who is not on a course of
orthodox medication, the practicalities of life often dictate
otherwise. While it is not an ideal situation, it is still worth
prescribing homoeopathically at home, especially if the
symptoms clearly suggest an obvious remedy. Although
antibiotics and other drugs may interfere with the effective
action of homoeopathic medicines, you don't need to worry
about orthodox medication and homoeopathic remedies
having an adverse toxic interaction with each other. This is
because homoeopathic medication works on the energy
levels of the patient, leaving no traceable chemical
constituents in the tissues or blood stream.

You can also consider taking your child to a homoeopathic
practitioner after the course of drugs has been completed,
especially if you feel your child is needing repeated courses of
conventional drugs for recurrent infections, such as colds,

sore throats, coughs or constant ear problems. If treatment is successful, you should find that homoeopathic help will enable your child to fight off illness more resiliently, resulting in fewer, and less severe, bouts of infection.

If you are considering prescribing homoeopathic medicines for your child and he is on a long-term course of orthodox drugs, such as steroids, never stop these drugs abruptly. There are many conventional treatments which require careful monitoring if they are to be reduced, and this should only be done with the full knowledge and co-operation of your GP.

How do I learn more about homoeopathic self-help?

If you are interested in learning more about homoeopathic prescribing at home, you will find attending a class in homoeopathic self-help of enormous value. These are held on a regular basis across the country and can be very valuable in creating an environment where you can compare notes with other beginners, or raise questions that have occurred to you while using this book.

If you would like more information about homoeopathic first-aid classes, contact your local library, education authority (extra-mural studies), local Homoeopathic Group, or Homoeopathic College.

How do I find a homoeopathic practitioner?

You can obtain registers of qualified homoeopathic practitioners from the following sources. The Society of Homoeopaths will supply you with a register of professional homoeopaths who have undergone a minimum of four years' training at an approved homoeopathic college. These are practitioners who are entitled to use the initials RS Hom.

If you require a list of orthodox doctors who also practice homoeopathy, you should contact The British Homoeopathic Association. These practitioners are entitled to use the initials MF Hom.

While registers are very useful in giving you a basic idea of qualifications held by individual practitioners in your area, the best method of finding a reputable homoeopath tends to be 'word of mouth'. In other words, if a friend's or relative's child has been treated by a practitioner they found professional, sympathetic, knowledgeable and sensitive to their needs, it would be worth enquiring further. Bear in mind that the relationship that develops between practitioner and patient will be unique, and what works for one individual may not work for another. Nevertheless, a strong personal recommendation can be of immense value in leading you in the right direction as you begin enquiries. Mothers of children at school or nursery, or teachers, can often be useful sources of information about local practitioners.

This method takes account of the fact that there are homoeopathic practitioners who trained before the college system was set up, and as a result, may not be included on available registers.

You can also consider looking through your local *Yellow Pages* entry under Homoeopathic Practitioners. This is not as good as a strong personal recommendation for the reasons given above, but if this is all that is available to you, look for the initials mentioned in the first two paragraphs.

If you feel your child has particular needs about which you are concerned, you can consider making a telephone enquiry.

This can provide you with an opportunity to discuss briefly the relevant issues with the practitioner's receptionist, or in some cases, directly with the homoeopath in person. This is also a useful way of finding out about practicalities, such as how long the initial consultation and follow-up appointments will be, and can also provide you with information about basic costs of treatment.

What should I expect if I take my child to a homoeopath?

The initial consultation with a homoeopath is a lengthy one: normally one or one and a half hours. However, the time spent will obviously depend on the age of your child. Taking the case notes for a baby who is a few weeks old will obviously take a shorter time than taking the case of a seven- or ten-year-old child.

The interview will be very thorough, with the homoeopath needing detailed information about the current problem, general health, current medication, medical history and as clear a sense as possible of the emotional and psychological characteristics of your child. If he is too young to communicate information himself, your homoeopath will need to gather as much information as possible from your perspective, plus any general observations made during the consultation. If your practitioner is also an orthodox doctor he or she might also want to conduct any appropriate physical examinations or tests.

If your child is old enough to communicate his or her own story, your homoeopath may want to spend time alone with him in order to establish a rapport. This can be immensely helpful in enabling the practitioner to gain a sense of the emotional and psychological characteristics of the patient.

It is often very helpful to take some of your child's favourite items along to the consultation, such as a cuddly toy, book or colouring set. Although many homoeopaths provide children's toys in their surgeries, bringing something from home serves an important dual function in giving your child something to do while the consultation is in progress, while also providing the security of a familiar object in unfamiliar surroundings.

After taking your child's case, the practitioner will analyse the information as a whole, and prescribe a homoeopathic remedy that is the closest match to the symptoms presented by your child. This is often given as a single tablet, or a short course of tablets, that may be taken daily. After you have observed your child's reaction to the remedy and communicated this to your practitioner, a decision will be made whether to wait, repeat the remedy or change the prescription. You will probably need to return with your child for repeat appointments every four or six weeks for the first few months in order for your practitioner to assess your child's progress.

KEYNOTES

Please refer back to the section in Homoeopathy in Action (on page 18) on how to use the following keynotes.

Aconite

Especially indicated for early stage of illness (first twenty-four – forty-eight hours) where there is feverishness and restlessness; especially if problems follow exposure to cold, dry winds, or a severe emotional trauma. Also well indicated for the fear and foreboding that may precede going into hospital for surgery.

Mental Picture
- Terribly anxious and fearful to the point of panic: child is convinced that he is going to die.
- Symptoms may emerge after shock or emotional trauma.
- Terrific sensitivity on mental, emotional and physical levels.
- Pains are unbearable, with aversion to being touched.

Fever
- Sudden onset of feverishness with hot head and cold body.
- Fever often follows on from exposure to dry, cold winds.
- High temperature often follows on from being chilled.

Head
- Sudden onset of headache with fever and shivering.
- Headaches or giddiness may follow an upsetting or frightening experience.

Eyes
- Sensitivity to light with redness, burning and watery eyes.
- Eye symptoms may develop rapidly and with severity.
- Often indicated for injuries to the eye with swelling and burning sensations.

Ears
- Earache of sudden onset after being exposed to chills or dry, cold winds.
- Hypersensitive to noise with severe pains in ears.
- Screams in panic and distress with pains.

Nose and Throat
- Clear, hot nasal discharge that is brought on suddenly by exposure to cold.
- Nose feels better for being out of doors in the fresh air.
- Dry, hoarse tingling throat and difficulty swallowing.
- Pain and constricted feeling on swallowing.

Chest
- Croupy cough which may be brought on by cold air or by being frightened.
- Wakes early in the night with violent cough and choking fits.
- Cough is aggravated by talking, eating, drinking, being upset or during the night.

Digestion
- Everything tastes bitter except water.
- Sudden onset of stomach upsets with marked thirst for water.
- Very tender around stomach region which is made worse by moving.
- Sudden appearance of diarrhoea with marked restlessness.

Sleep
- May be drowsy during the day and sleepless at night.
- Disturbed sleep with terrors and nightmares.
- Tosses and turns in sleep.

Skin
- Extra sensitive skin with the least touch causing discomfort.

Worse from
- Extreme changes of temperature
- Warm, airless rooms
- Night
- Lying on the painful side

Better for
- Fresh air
- Undisturbed sleep
- Sweating

Allium cepa

Mental Picture
- Very sensitive to pain.
- Anxious or withdrawn, with catarrh.

Head
- Dull headache with head cold that gets worse in the evening and in warm rooms. Pain feels better in fresh, open air.

Eyes
- Eyes run with bland tears.
- Left eye may be more affected than right.
- Eyes feel sensitive and are badly affected by bright light.
- Swelling around margins of eyes with itching, burning and irritation.

Nose
- Very runny nose which burns the upper lip: eyes and nose run at the same time.
- Violent sneezing that is set off when in contact with pollen.

Chest
- Tickling in throat which sets off cough.
- Sneezing with coughing which can be made worse by inhaling cold air.
- Tightness in chest is worse each evening.

Worse from
Warm rooms
Evenings
Rest

Better for
Open, fresh air
Cold in general

Antimonium crudum

Symptoms may follow from being chilled after cool bathing, or from exposure to cold air. Exhaustion and prostration accompany most symptoms.

Mental Picture
- Dislike of being approached or questioned.
- Easily made irritable and angry or sulky.
- Rejects advances with temper.

Fever
- Very chilled without thirst, followed by heat and perspiration with desire to drink.
- Sweats on exertion and at night.

Head
- Headaches from being chilled or from upset stomach.

Eyes
- Sore eyes which are very sensitive to light.
- Intense itching of eyes with inflamed lids which stick together at night.

Ears
- Sensations of heat in ears with shooting pains.
- Temporary difficulty in hearing, with buzzing sounds in ear.

Nose and Throat
- Sore nostrils with crusting.
- Nasal obstruction which is worse in a warm room or at night.

Chest
- Cough which is made worse by entering a warm room.
- Initial bout of coughing is the most severe, with succeeding bouts becoming less intense.
- Burning sensation in chest with coughing spasms.

Digestion
- Full feelings in the stomach which are not relieved by vomiting or bringing up wind.
- Bloating of stomach with burning sensations.
- Nocturnal, watery diarrhoea which may be brought on by becoming chilled after being overheated.
- Diarrhoea alternating with constipation.

Skin
- Prickly heat which is aggravated by exercise.
- Eruptions are very itchy and have a bluish tinge.

Worse from
Heat
Being chilled
Night
Being touched

Better from
Keeping still
Lying down

Antimonium tartaricum

L ess likely to be indicated in the early stage of illness:
most often needed in the established phase where
symptoms have developed insidiously.

Mental Picture
- Very irritable, anxious and restless.
- Every effort is exhausting: just can't be bothered.
- Although unhappy about receiving attention, child likes being carried.
- May be clingy.

Fever
- Chilly, pale and cold to the touch.
- Very clammy and sweaty.
- Although so chilly, child complains if room is over-heated, or if too warmly wrapped up.

Head
- Sensation of dullness and drowsiness.
- May be confused.

Eyes
- Must keep eyes closed because of discomfort.
- Tired and bruised feelings in eyes.

Nose and Throat
- May have nose bleeds with productive nasal discharge.
- Very sensitive air passages to change to wet weather.
- Productive catarrh in throat.

Chest
- Lots of mucus in the chest which is difficult to raise.
- Rattling and bubbling in chest from accumulation of mucus.
- Cough is worse in the early morning, from eating and getting angry.
- Wakes from sleep unable to breathe from congestion in chest.
- Repeated attacks of bronchitis in children.

Digestion
- Lots of saliva which accumulates in the mouth.
- Tongue coated with white fur.
- Severe nausea which is relieved by vomiting.
- Sharp, colicky pains with diarrhoea.
- Cold sweat and exhaustion with vomiting and diarrhoea.

Sleep
- Very drowsy after vomiting.
- Child is confused and giddy on waking.

Skin
- Large, bluish coloured eruptions which leave bluish-red marks when healed.

Worse from
Change to damp, cold weather
Cold bathing
Evenings
Lying down

Better for
Bringing up phlegm
Sitting up
Bringing up wind
Cool air

Apis

Mental Picture
- Very fussy, fidgety and irritable.
- Hypersensitive to least contact or touch.
- Problems may follow stress or emotional upset.

Fever
- Absence of thirst with high temperature.
- Thirst appears once high fever has subsided and child may complain of feeling chilled.
- Desire for coolness and aversion to heat in any form.

Head
- Hot, throbbing pains with headache.
- Headache worse for warm rooms and jolting.

Eyes
- Tremendous puffing and swelling of eyelids: lids below the eyes swell like water bags.
- Sensitivity to light with watering of the eyes.
- Bathing the eyes in cool water is temporarily soothing.

Nose and Throat
- Violent sneezing with blocked nostrils and scanty nasal discharge.

- Swelling of the throat with puffy uvula: may look water-logged.
- Difficulty swallowing because of swelling: even taking a sip of water is difficult.
- Throat feels constricted.

Chest
- Suffocative feelings in a warm room.
- Difficult breathing made worse by leaning forwards or backwards.

Digestion
- Swelling and tension in region of stomach which is sensitive to touch.
- Burning pains in stomach which are made worse by sneezing.
- Raw, burning anus after diarrhoea: pains are relieved by bathing in cool water.

Sleep
- Restless and cries in sleep.
- Constantly moving around bed at night in search of a cool spot.
- May throw covers off in an effort to cool down.

Skin
- Pink, puffy swellings that look as though water is trapped beneath the skin.
- Stinging and itching sensations with eruptions that are much relieved by cool bathing, and made markedly worse by exposure to warmth in any form.
- Often indicated for hives that result from becoming over heated.

Worse from
Heat in any form: fire, bathing, or stuffy rooms
Touch
Lying down
After sleep
At night

Better for
Cool in any form: cool air, applications or uncovering
Walking about
Sitting up

Arnica

The first remedy to consider where there has been bruising, shock or trauma of any kind.

Mental Picture
- Wants to be left alone during immediate shock following an accident: pushes people away.
- Because pains are so strong, dislikes anyone approaching because of an aversion to being touched.
- Irritability with pain.

Head
- Giddiness after waking or walking, which is worse closing the eyes.
- One-sided headache with nausea.

Eyes
- Bruising or bleeding following injury.
- Eye-strain or conjunctivitis with burning sensations.

Ears

- Loss of hearing or hearing only muffled sounds after an injury.
- Shooting pains in, or about, the ears.

Nose and Throat

- Nose bleed follows tingling in nose, or injury.
- Bruised, aching feeling in throat.

Chest

- Stitching pains in the chest which are made worse by movement and coughing.
- Cough is dry and tickly and worse in the morning.
- Child cries before coughing bout.

Digestion

- Nausea with excessive amount of saliva.
- Colicky pains in the abdomen with accompanying wind.
- Diarrhoea passed involuntarily.

Sleep

- Extremely restless with the bed seeming too hard.
- Complains of aching all over with tiredness.
- Inability to get to sleep, due to over-tiredness.
- Difficulty getting to sleep until early morning: once asleep, wakes from bad dreams.

Skin

- Bruising with tenderness and aching soreness.
- Boils which have not yet come to a head but which are very painful.

- Generalised aching, throbbing and burning pains with exhausted sensation.
- Restless with aching.

Worse from
Damp
Cold
Movement
Being touched

Better for
Lying undisturbed with head lower than body

Arsenicum album

Mental Picture
- Very anxious and prostrated with illness.
- Extremely physically and mentally restless.
- Over-sensitive and fussy about everything.
- Terrible anxiety leading to panic that gets worse as the night goes on.
- Feels much worse for being alone.

Fever
- Terribly chilly with fever, with ice-cold sensations surging through body.
- May feel as though burning up from head to feet: sensation is relieved by warm applications.
- When feverish, there is a thirst for sips of warm drinks rather than a large amount in one gulp.

Head

- Nausea and possible vomiting with headache.
- The head is the only part of the body that is relieved by exposure to cool, fresh air.
- Headaches often come on at night or in the afternoon and get steadily worse as the night goes on.

Eyes

- Great sensitivity to light with redness of the eyes and burning sensations.
- Swelling of upper and lower lids.
- Discomfort in the eyes is relieved by warmth.

Nose and Throat

- Violent sneezing with scanty, clear nasal discharge.
- Runny nose leaves the nostrils and upper lip red and sore.
- Burning pains in the throat which are soothed by warm drinks.

Chest

- Dry cough which is worse at night and better for sitting propped up in bed.
- Wheezy and anxious with coughing spasms.
- Cough is made worse by lying down, eating or being out of doors.
- Asthmatic symptoms often brought on by panic or stress.

Digestion

- Burning pains in stomach which are relieved by warm drinks and warm applications.
- Vomiting and diarrhoea occur together with exhaustion and restlessness.

- Sips of warm drinks are tolerated, but cold drinks are vomited back immediately.

Sleep
- Drowsy by day and sleepless at night.
- Very restless at night when all symptoms are aggravated.
- May refuse to stay in bed from restlessness and wants to wander about.

Skin
- Very itchy, burning skin that is made much worse from scratching.
- Scratching may be intense enough to cause bleeding and weeping of the skin.
- After rubbing, the itching feels temporarily better, but the burning remains.
- Eruptions feel better for warmth.

Worse from
Cold in any form
After midnight
Being alone
Draughts
Lying flat in bed

Better for
Warmth in any form
Sitting propped up in bed
Company
Headaches are better for fresh air.

Belladonna

L ike Aconite, this remedy is most often required for the early stage of illness, especially when symptoms have been rapid and violent in onset. For later, more established stages of illness, another remedy is likely to be indicated.

Mental Picture
- Very irritable and bad-tempered with illness.
- Children who are normally placid and easy to please become difficult and very touchy when ill.
- Easily over-excitable which can lead to drowsiness and lethargy.
- Very adversely affected by stimulation of any kind such as noise, light and movement.
- May hallucinate with high temperature.
- More irritable than anxious or fearful.

Fever
- Rapid onset of high fever with very dry, hot, red skin.
- Although very hot with fever, feels worse for cold in general.
- High temperature may result in hot head with cold extremeties.
- Sweats on parts of the body that are covered.
- Very rapid pulse with fever.

Head
- Violent headaches with very sensitive scalp: refuses to have hair touched.
- May feel more comfortable bending head backwards.
- Contrary to general features of the remedy, headaches

may be relieved by open air and cool applications.
- Head pain is much worse from bending forwards, lying flat, bright light and jarring.

Eyes
- Pupils become dilated with high temperature.
- Eyes feel hot and look very inflamed and red.
- Twitching and spasmodic movement of eyelids.

Ears
- Earache of sudden, violent onset: often brought on by exposure to cold.
- Ear pain is often right-sided.
- Hearing becomes painfully acute with over-sensitivity to voices.

Nose and Throat
- Red, swollen tip to nose as well as generally red, flushed face.
- Very acute sense of smell with nasty odour in nose.
- Very painful, throbbing, dry throat with difficulty swallowing.
- Sits forward in order to swallow liquids.
- Tonsils may be very inflamed especially on the right side.
- Rapid hoarseness or complete loss of voice.

Chest
- Dry, barking cough which is made worse by lying down at night, crying, and on breathing in deeply.
- Relieved temporarily if mucus can be expelled.
- Irritating tickling in throat precedes coughing fit.

Digestion
- Cramping, colicky pains in stomach and abdomen, which feel better for bending forwards or backwards.
- Stomach and abdomen are hypersensitive to touch of bed covers or clothing.
- Diarrhoea with constant desire to go.

Sleep
- Very restless, twitchy and disturbed sleep.
- Jerks awake on falling asleep, or wakes with a start after a nightmare.
- Talks or moans in sleep.
  Although very drowsy, cannot fall into refreshing sleep.

Skin
- Very dry, red skin that it so intensely flushed it radiates heat.
- Skin is very painful and hypersensitive to touch.
- One of the first remedies to think of in cases of sunburn.

Worse from
Stimulation of any kind
Lying on painful parts
Cold and draughts

Better for
Resting undisturbed
Lying propped up in bed
Warm, quiet, dark rooms
Bending head backwards

Bryonia

Often indicated for symptoms that have shown a slow, insidious development.

Mental Picture

- Very irritable and cross when disturbed.
- Discontented and difficult to please: asks for something and then rejects it.
- Child cries and complains she wants to go home when she is in her own bed.
- Wants to lie still in a quiet room: strong aversion to making any kind of effort.

Fever

- Very thirsty for large quantities of cold drinks, with high temperature.
- Aversion to being in a warm room or being too well-wrapped up.
- Sweaty with fever, especially at night.

Head

- Severe frontal headache which is worse for movement of any kind, especially stooping.
- Headache often occurs as the result of constipation.
- Pain is worse for heat and better for cool applications.

Eyes

- Sore, sensitive eyes feel worse for slightest movement.
- Eyes feel hot and gritty.

Nose and Throat
- Nasal discharge with pains in forehead.
- Red, sore swelling of nose.
- Generalised dryness of air passages with irritation being felt in the throat and upper chest.
- Mucus is scanty and difficult to raise.

Chest
- Dry, irritating, tickly cough with possible gagging.
- Coughing spasms are often brought on by entering a warm atmosphere.
- Wants to take a deep breath but this aggravates the cough.
- Pain in chest which is relieved by firm pressure, so child holds or presses hand to painful area in chest or head when coughing.

Digestion
- Very dry mouth with marked thirst.
- Eating and movement make nausea much worse.
- Sick feeling temporarily relieved by belching.
- Draws legs up to abdomen with colicky pains.
- Exhausting diarrhoea that is made much worse by moving about.
- Diarrhoea may be brought on by eating acid fruit.
- When constipation is present, stools are characteristically dry, large, hard, dark in colour and very difficult to pass.

Sleep
- Very drowsy during the day with great difficulty sleeping at night.

- Unrefreshing sleep with a tendency to wake in fright when dropping off to sleep.

Worse from
Warmth in general
Physical or mental effort
Sitting up
Moving about, especially after resting

Better for
Resting
Lying still
Firm pressure to painful area
Perspiring
Cold in general

Calc carb

This is a remedy which is seldom indicated for short-lived, acute problems, and most often used for long-term, 'constitutional' treatment. Therefore, it is a remedy that does not require frequent repetition.

Mental Picture
- Strong-willed, obstinate children who approach tasks with dogged determination at their own pace: dislike being hurried.
- Poor long-term stamina: exhaustion can set in rapidly.
- Sensitive children who are full of fears, such as darkness, being alone, or other people seeing their confusion or distress.
- Clingy children who react very badly to criticism.
- Child may appear withdrawn or slow. Developmental

milestones such as closure of fontanelles, teething and walking happen more slowly than expected.

Fever
- Children requiring Calc carb are subject to repeated infections in winter, such as colds, coughs, sore throats, swollen glands and ear infections.
- Although complaining of flushes of heat, extremities feel cold, sweaty and excessively clammy.
- When feverish, sudden sweats may occur from exertion.
- Generally sweaty, especially on head and feet in bed at night.

Head
- Sick headache which is relieved by warmth and aggravated by colds and draughts.
- Pain generally relieved by resting.

Eyes
- Eyes are easily fatigued with a resulting filmy or veiled sensation.
- Rapid straining of eye muscles from reading or watching television.

Ears
- Chronic ear infections with swelling of glands in winter.
- Stubborn catarrh resulting in hearing difficulties.

Nose and Throat
- Thick nasal discharge with soreness of nose.
- Recurrent winter sore throats with swollen glands.
- Painless hoarseness or loss of voice on waking.

Chest
- Tickly cough at night or rattly cough with large amounts of thick, yellow mucus which tastes sweet.

Digestion
- Slow digestion with a tendency to stubborn constipation or alternation between diarrhoea and constipation.
- Food cravings include eggs, pasta, bread, sweets and salt. Child may try to eat chalk or coal.
- Dislike of hot dishes, milk or slimy foods.
- Child feels better when constipated.

Sleep
- Disturbed sleep with tendencies to recurrent nightmares. Child wakes from sleep so upset it is very difficult to calm or pacify him.
- Grinds teeth in sleep or sleepwalks.

Skin
- May be generally dry and chaps or cracks easily in winter.
- Tendencies to chronic skin conditions such as eczema, nappy rash, and cradle cap.

Worse from
Cold and wet
Draughts
Changes from warm to cold weather

Better for
Warmth
Dry weather
When constipated

Calc phos

O ften indicated for fractures that refuse to knit, or
problems associated with teething.

Mental Picture
- Generally nervy, timid and sensitive.
- Irritable and wants to be left alone.
- Contrary: when out of doors wants to be in, and when indoors wants to be out.
- Illness often follows emotional strain or shock.

Fever
- Generally chilly and suffers from the cold.
- Sweats a lot at night.

Head
- Dull headache after school or from watching television, which is worse for any physical effort, better for being quiet.
- Headache may also come on after exposure to cold winds involving the whole head.

Eyes
- Very sensitive to light with desire to rub the eye all the time.
- Constant sense of something in the eye which is irritating.

Ears
- Earache from cold weather, with irritating discharge.
- Noises in the ear with pain.

Nose and Throat

- Runny nose in a cold room, stuffed up in a warm atmosphere.
- Nose bleeds from blowing the nose.
- Swollen and sore nostrils.
- Chronically enlarged tonsils with constricted feeling in throat.
- Lots of coughing up of mucus which settles in throat.

Chest

- Dry cough which is preceded by hoarseness in cold weather.
- Lots of rattly mucus in the chest which is very difficult to raise.
- Coughing is relieved by lying down.

Digestion

- Bad taste in the mouth.
- Vomiting and colic after every feed in babies which is better for belching and passing wind.
- Watery diarrhoea or greenish-coloured stools that appear during teething.
- Teeth are very soft when they emerge and full of cavities.

Sleep

- Sleep may be disturbed from growing pains.
- Sleepless around midnight.
- Difficulty coming round in the morning.

Skin

- Eczema often affects the external ear in children: general area looks very swollen.

Worse from
Cold and wet
Change of weather to winter
Cold winds
Effort of any kind

Better for
Dry, warm weather
Warm bathing
Resting

Calendula

Mainly used as an external application in the form of lotion, cream, ointment or diluted tincture. The antiseptic properties of Calendula make it an ideal skin salve for wounds and abrasions, since it promotes healing of skin, slows down bleeding and inhibits infection.

Carbo veg

Especially indicated for general symptoms of shock.

Mental Picture
- Apathetic and indifferent.
- Irritability.
- Confusion and withdrawal.
- Anxious and afraid of the dark.

Fever
- Chilly, clammy and sweaty with strong desire for fresh air: asks to be fanned.
- Pale with bluish tinge to skin.
- Although cold on the surface, may feel burning hot inside, especially in the chest

Head
- Headache with throbbing in temples or sensation of a tight band around the head.
- Pains are worse from movement and effort.

Eyes
- Burning pains in eyes with heavy, itchy edges to lids.

Ears
- Noises and stuffed up sensations in ears.
- Chronic ear pains with a watery, burning, smelly discharge.

Nose and Throat
- Sneezing with tendency to frequent nose bleeds.
- Feels generally unwell with nasal mucus which is made worse by extremes of temperature.
- Nose feels cold and goes red and sore at the tip.
- Burning sensations in the throat which lead to hoarseness.
- Pains in throat are worse from talking, clearing the throat and damp air.

Chest

- Coughing spasms often end in gagging or vomiting with flushing of the face.
- Suffocating sensations come on after lying down and are relieved by contact with fresh air.
- Rattling mucus in the chest which is very difficult to raise.
- Sensations of weakness and burning in the chest causing great distress.

Digestion

- Nausea and general queasiness from over eating.
- Constant belching which gives temporary relief.
- Burning sensations in the stomach.
- Colicky pains with rumbling and diarrhoea.

Sleep

- Twitches and jerks in sleep.
- Wakes covered in perspiration.

Worse from

Warmth
Stuffy atmospheres
Humidity
Cold
Movement
After eating

Better for

Fresh air
Being fanned
After sleep
Belching

Chamomilla

Mental Picture
- Child screams and howls with frustration and pain.
- Nothing will pacify child apart from being rocked or carried around.
- Throws toys to the ground in anger because of pain.
- Impatience and extreme irritability: may bang head against the wall in desperation.
- Physically and emotionally over-sensitive.
- Aversion to being touched.

Fever
- General flushed appearance: sometimes one cheek looks red and the other pale.
- Thirsty for cold water.
- Warm head which is moist with sweat.
- Due to feeling hot, infant's feet are constantly on the move in bed in search of a cool spot.

Head
- Headache brought on by, or made worse from, anger
- Pain is better for heat and wrapping up.

Eyes
- Eyes swollen on waking with lids that stick together.

Ears
Severe ear pains that are worse on bending forward, which causes cries of pain.

Nose and Throat
- Blocked nose with hot, watery discharge.
- Lots of dry sneezing.

Chest
- Hacking, dry cough at night, also set off by talking.
- Cough disturbs sleep and leaves child feeling bad-tempered on waking.
- Anger or tantrums may bring on a coughing fit.

Digestion
- Green watery stools caused by teething which smell like rotten eggs.
- Colicky pains which are not relieved by passing wind, but which feel better for warmth applied locally.
- Infant doubles up bringing knees up to chest and screams with pain.

Sleep
Sleep is disturbed with tossing, moaning and starting.

Worse from
Exposure to heat and draughts
Windy and wet weather
First part of the night

Better for
Moist, warm, humid conditions
Being rocked or carried

Colocynthis

Mental Picture
- Pains may be preceded by anger, frustration, irritability or grief.
- Child writhes about in pain and anguish: may double up in order to get relief.
- Quite unable to keep still because of extreme discomfort. Screams with rage and pain.
- Baby or infant instinctively lies on belly, since pressure relieves pain.
- Onset and relief of symptoms are both abrupt.

Fever
Chilly with marked sensitivity to cold, especially damp cold. Constant thirst with hot, dry skin.

Head
- One-sided neuralgic pains in face which come in waves.
- Discomfort is eased by pressure and warm applications.

Eyes
Sharp pains in eyes that are better from pressure.

Nose, Throat and Chest
- Very runny nose in the mornings without sneezing.
- Tightness of chest with dry, irritating cough.

Digestion
- Very heavily coated white tongue.
- Lots of windy bloating with strong colicky pains that are made much worse by eating or drinking.

- Pains may be accompanied by vomiting, diarrhoea and a lot of wind being passed.
- Colicky pains are temporarily relieved by infant lying on belly or drawing knees up: also reacts well to warmth.
- As soon as anything is eaten, diarrhoea begins again.

Worse from
Keeping still
Cold: especially cold and damp
Eating fruit
Drinking iced drinks when over heated

Better for
Locally applied heat
Bending double
Firm pressure
Passing wind or stool

Dioscorea

Mental Picture
- Weepy, irritable and cross
- Lethargic and exhausted

Head
- Headache with colicky pains in abdomen or head cold.
- Pains in forehead that extend to nose, with sick feeling.

Nose and throat
- Lots of sneezing with watery discharge from nose.
- Burning and smarting in throat with sick feelings on swallowing.
- Tight feelings in throat with swollen glands.

Chest

- Spasms of coughing with pain in area of belly button; headache.
- Coughing begins by tickling low in throat.

Digestion

- Constant distress and discomfort in stomach and abdomen with colicky pains that come every few minutes.
- Pains are aggravated by pressure of clothes or covers and made easier by stretching out (the opposite of Chamomilla).
- Constant need to move with flitting pains.
- Terrible twisting, cramping pains before passing a bowel movement.

Sleep

- Symptoms are generally worse after sleep.
- Goes to sleep late from discomfort and wakes early.
- Moves constantly in sleep even though it hurts.

Worse from
Early morning
On waking
Touch

Better for
Stretching out
Open air
Moving about

Euphrasia

Head
Headache with accompanying severe eye symptoms.

Eyes
- Eyes are severely affected with terrible sensitivity to sunlight, and burning tears that hurt the eyes and make the cheeks look irritated.
- Margins of eyelids look red and swollen and feel as though they are burning.
- Child wants to rub the eyes constantly because they are so irritated.
- Lids stick together by morning from discharge which is secreted overnight.

Nose
- Runny nose with bland nasal discharge which is fluent in the morning and when outside.

Chest
- Loose cough with nose and eye symptoms.

Worse from
Windy weather
Cold air
In the morning
Bright light
Warmth

Better for
Darkness

Ferrum phos

Often indicated for early stages of inflammatory illness where symptoms do not have the terror of Aconite or the violence and hyperirritability of Belladonna.

Mental Picture
- Mentally and physically sluggish.
- Feels weak and is easily exhausted: child may appear indifferent to things that would normally be of interest.
- Symptoms may appear after exposure to cold or loss of fluids, such as sweating or bleeding from an injury.
- Flushes easily when excited.

Fever
- Generally chilly and sensitive to open air.
- Face flushes readily with fever.

Head
- Headache which is relieved by nose bleed.
- Face flushes with headache and general sensitivity of scalp.

Nose and Throat
- Regular nose bleeds in children.
- Sore, swollen throat on waking which is worse on swallowing saliva.
- Throat is generally dry, red and painful.

Chest
- Hoarse voice with catarrh of throat.
- Painful cough with rattling mucus in chest.

- Cough brought on by touching external throat or by bending over.
- Cough is easier indoors.

Digestion
- Very poor appetite with nausea.
- Very thirsty for drinks of water.
- Sick headache.

Sleep
- Drowsiness and indifference by day.
- Very restless at night with distress on waking.
- Unable to sleep because of pains.

Worse from
Eating
Moving
At night
Open air
Being touched
Cold

Better for
Gentle movement
Rest

Gelsemium

Indicated for classic 'flu symptoms that take days to develop, rather than abrupt onset of illness.

Mental Picture
- Mentally and physically fatigued, weary and exhausted.
- Doesn't want to be bothered with anything; just wants to be left alone.
- Can't make the effort to get involved with anything that requires any enthusiasm or effort.
- Child may feel afraid in the dark and ask for a night light.
- Symptoms may be preceded by excitement, sudden fright or bad news.

Fever
- Muscle weakness and trembling with fever: legs feel wobbly.
- Face and head may be hot and flushed, with cold extremeties.
- Dislike of being in a hot room despite shivers and chills that run up and down spine.
- Lots of sweating which does not relieve symptoms.

Head
- Headache with dizziness and unsteadiness which is worse on waking.
- Characteristic feeling as though head was compressed by a tight band above the eyes, with sore scalp and tight neck and shoulder muscles.
- Headaches feel worse for warmth and better for lying still propped up in bed.

Eyes
- Eyelids look heavy and droopy with tiredness.
- Sore eyes with blurred vision and dizziness that are made worse by movement.

Nose and Throat

- Slow-developing cold symptoms that begin with severe sneezing bouts, with hot nasal discharge.
- Nose feels completely blocked and nostrils may get very red and sore.
- Sore throat looks red, puffy and swollen, and pains shoot from the throat to the ear on swallowing.
- Child complains of difficulty swallowing due to a lump in the throat.

Chest

- Violent coughing spasms with sore chest.
- Sudden bouts of breathlessness with shallow breathing.

Digestion

- Dry lips and mouth with no thirst.
- Painless diarrhoea from anticipation or 'nerves'.
- Withdrawn with nervous diarrhoea rather than talkative.

Sleep

- Sweaty and disturbed during sleep with aches and pains.
- Wakes suddenly with a jerk from rest.

Worse from

Hot rooms
Wet weather
Direct sunlight
Cold draught

Better for

Open, fresh air
After sweating or passing water
Warmth

Hepar sulph

Mental Picture
- Terribly sensitive with a tendency to outbursts of irritability.
- Gets furious very quickly and is generally very difficult to please or get on with.
- Child may get violent with temper and frustration.
- Unable to stand pain or physical discomfort.

Fever
- Sweats easily and profusely from the least effort: perspiration may have a nasty odour.
- Hypersensitive to cold air and draughts: must be kept completely and snuggly covered or feels terrible.

Eyes
- Styes or conjunctivitis with thick, sticky, yellow discharge.
- Extreme sensitivity to light.

Ears
- Earache with thick, yellowish, offensive-smelling discharge.
- Right ear more likely to be affected than left.

Nose and Throat
- Sneezing from least contact with cold air.
- Possible sinus involvement with thick, yellow, nasty-smelling mucus which causes pressure at the root of the nose.
- Sore throat with sensation as though a fish bone were lodged in sides of throat.

- Very inflamed or septic tonsils with yellow-coloured ulceration.
- Laryngitis which is much worse for exposure to cold.

Chest
- Severe cough which is aggravated by contact with cold air, or by uncovering body.
- Lots of rattling mucus in chest which is very difficult to dislodge.
- Feels sick and sweats copiously trying to bring up mucus from chest.
- Throat and chest feel better for warm drinks.

Digestion
- Lots of belching with swelling and tension of stomach.
- Diarrhoea may be painless and brought on immediately after eating.

Sleep
- Drowsy during the day and very restless and sweaty at night.

Skin
- Skin is very slow to heal and the smallest cut seems to fester.
- Especially indicated for boils and pimples which are slow to come to a head, provided general symptoms agree.
- Wounds and eruptions are very sensitive to contact with cold air.

Worse from
Cold draughts
Cold food and drink
Light touch
Lying on the painful side
Morning and evening

Better for
Warmth in general
After a meal
Warm, wet weather

Hypericum

This remedy has a particular affinity for injured areas that are rich in nerve supply, e.g. crushed fingers or toes.

Mental Picture
• Drowsiness or sadness and distress following injury.

Head
• Headaches may follow a fall involving the base of the spine.

General features
• Crushing pains in fingers, toes or base of spine after injury, with terrific sensitivity to touch.
• Injured areas are so sensitive that any movement results in distress and crying.
• Pain is especially bad on rising from sitting.
• Darting and intermittent pains shoot away from injured area.

Worse from
Cold, damp air
Touch
Movement

Better for
Keeping still

Ignatia

Mental Picture
- Especially indicated in times of emotional distress and grief, especially in children who are sensitive, nervous or excitable.
- May bottle up emotions until they explode in trembling or hysterical crying.
- Often helpful in easing symptoms of homesickness where there is a great deal of distress.
- Contradictory moods: laughter alternates with weeping, or anger with remorse.
- Child feels misunderstood and resentful.
- Generally sensitive to pain, noise or criticism.
- Constant sighing.

Head
- Headache brought on by stress, grief or exposure to strong smells.

Nose and Throat
- Strong sensation of a lump in the throat which makes swallowing difficult.

- Constant soreness of throat or loss of voice since emotional upset.

Digestion
- Bitter taste in the mouth with lots of saliva.
- Belching and hiccoughing which are worse from eating.
- Spasmodic pains in stomach with constipated feeling.
- Soft stools are harder to pass than hard ones.
- Painless diarrhoea from emotional distress.

Sleep
- Jerks and twitches in light sleep: wakes very readily.
- Limbs jerk on going to sleep.
- Whimpering in sleep.

Worse from
Eating sweets
Emotional upset or shock
Strong odours
Pressure on non-painful areas
Yawning

Better for
Warmth
Eating
Being distracted
Pressure to painful parts

Ipecac

Mental Picture
- Very impatient and full of dissatisfaction.
- Child screams and cries at least provocation.
- Very sensitive to noise, especially loud music.

Fever
- Exceptionally chilly with the least draught causing discomfort.
- Cold shivers and trembling.
- Thirstless although feverish.
- Onset of symptoms may be sudden.

Head
- Sick headache which involves the whole head.
- Child looks deathly pale and is sick with headache.

Eyes
- Sensitivity to light with pains and watering in the eye.

Nose and Throat
- Blocked nose with easy nose bleeds.
- When nose runs, mucus may be blood-streaked.

Chest
- Dry, irritating cough from tickling in air passages.
- Coughing spasms come on suddenly with lots of wheezing and rattling in chest.
- Bouts of coughing cause gagging and often end in vomiting.

- Breathing difficulties result in child sitting up to catch breath.
- Child may go pale and bluish when coughing spasms are severe, especially in cases of whooping cough.

Digestion

- Terrible, persistent, deathly nausea accompanies all symptoms.
- Sick feeling is not relieved by vomiting.
- Abdomen may feel swollen and tender with constant desire to pass stools.
- Diarrhoea in infants may be green in colour and foamy.

Worse from
Cold or great heat
Eating

Better for
Firm pressure
Fresh air
Closing eyes

Kali bich

Mental Picture

- Listless and lethargic.
- Unwilling to do anything that requires mental or physical effort.
- Dislikes meeting new people.

Head

- Migraine-type headache which causes nausea and vomiting which is worse at night.

- Sinusitis with pain at the root of the nose.

Eyes
- Eyes burn and itch with sensitivity to light.
- Edges of eyelids become red and swollen.
- Chronic conjunctivitis with heat and redness of the eyeball.

Ears
- Earache with swollen glands.
- Chronic ear pain with yellow, offensive-smelling discharge.

Nose and Throat
- Catarrh at back of throat which is stubborn, stringy and difficult to raise.
- Child complains of an irritating sensation as though a hair is resting on the back of the tongue.
- Nose blocked from yellow, sticky discharge.
- Sore throat with swollen, water-logged uvula.
- Sore throat soothed by warm drinks.

Chest
- Croupy cough with gagging and breathlessness in an effort to raise sticky mucus.
- Cough is worse on waking in the morning and may be accompanied by back pain. It is eased by lying down and warmth.
- If coughing occurs after eating, food is vomited back up.
- Wakes complaining of pressure on chest which is relieved by bringing up mucus.

Digestion
- Stomach upsets accompany headaches and are worse for eating.
- Feels better for belching.
- Stubborn constipation with headache and lethargy.
- Pale stools may be passed involuntarily.

Sleep
- Very drowsy and unrefreshed by sleep: wakes with a jump around 2 a.m. from breathlessness, nausea or feeling hot and sweaty. Exhausted through the day as a result.

Worse from
Winter weather
Cold winds
Touch
Stooping
Waking from sleep

Better for
Warmth
Lying in bed
Movement
Firm pressure
Summer weather

Kali carb

Mental Picture
- Highly-strung, edgy and irritable from over-tiredness.
- Jumpy and over-sensitive to noise or shocks of any kind.
- Lots of fears: including a fear of being alone and of ghosts.
- Full of complaints and feels at odds with everyone.

Head

- Burning pains in scalp or sinuses above eyes and in cheeks.
- Pains are much worse for contact with cold air, so child feels more comfortable from having head well wrapped up.

Eyes

- Puffy swelling of eyelids with sharp pains in the eyes.

Ears

- Cracking sensations in ears.

Nose and Throat

- Nasal passages feel uncomfortably dry and nose generally looks very red and swollen.
- Nose blocks up in a warm atmosphere which eases headache.
- Recurrent colds with loss of voice.
- Sticking pains or a sensation of swallowing over a lump or ball in the throat.

Chest

- Dry, hacking cough with swollen upper eyelids.
- Chilly feelings in chest with wheezing and vomiting.
- Chronic nasty-tasting catarrh may hang on from an attack of measles or other acute illness.
- Mucus is yellowish-green in colour, lumpy and difficult to raise.

Digestion
- Lots of bloating and swelling in abdomen which comes on after eating.
- Colicky pains that are relieved by warmth, hot drinks and hot water bottles. Pains feel better for bending double.
- Constipation or diarrhoea with burning in rectum and anus.

Sleep
- Wakes from horrible nightmares in the early hours and cannot get back to sleep again.

Worse from
Cold air and draughts
Change in weather
Least touch or pressure on painful part

Better for
Warm, moist weather
During the day
Leaning forward

Kali mur

Head
- Headache with vomiting of white mucus that looks like milk.

Eyes
- White mucus discharged from eyes or yellowy-green matter that becomes crusty. Eyes feel sandy or gritty.

Ears
- Chronic ear problems with deafness and swollen glands which hurt on swallowing.

Nose and Throat
- Thick white mucus with stuffed feeling in head. Frequent nose bleeds.
- Very swollen tonsils with stringy, white mucus which is very painful to swallow.

Chest
- Hard, harsh and croupy cough with loss of voice.

Digestion
- Refusal to eat with whitish-looking coating on tongue. Constipation or diarrhoea with pale, lightish-coloured stools. Diarrhoea may follow eating too many fatty foods.

Skin
- Scurfy, flaky eruptions on head and face. Skin may be so dry it looks as though it is coated with flour.

Worse from
Motion
Warmth of bed
Rising in the morning
Rich or fatty foods

Kreosotum

Mental Picture
- Tearful over minor things and very difficult to satisfy.
- Irritable with pain and very restless.
- Nervous and excitable.

Fever
- Very chilly generally with cold legs and feet, but hot face.
- Intense, burning thirst.

Head
- Drowsy with throbbing, bursting headache.
- Scalp sensitive to touch.

Eyes
- Eyelids inflamed and sore with hot, burning tears.

Ears
- Red, hot, burning, itchy ears with swollen glands and stiff neck.
- Deafness with noises in ears.

Nose and Throat
- Offensive discharge from nose with well-established catarrh.
- Dry, burning throat which feels worse for swallowing.

Chest
- Difficulty taking a deep breath because of sense of fullness in chest.
- Breathing worse in a warm room and better in open air.

- Burning pains in chest with wheezing or retching, especially in morning.
- Cough every winter.

Stomach

- Teething with screaming, distress and restlessness.
- Teeth are of very poor quality and have black marks as they come through the gums.
- Gums are sensitive, spongy and bleed easily.
- Burning in stomach with belching.
- Children scream and strain on passing a stool.

Sleep

- Lies awake at night tossing and turning and yawning.
- Child may moan in sleep, or doze with eyes half open.

Skin

- Burning, itching skin that is much worse in the evening and at night. Moist, itchy eczema on face that causes restlessness.

Worse from
Out of doors
Cold air and washing
Resting
Touch
At night

Better for
Warmth
Movement
Pressure

Lachesis

Mental Picture
- Anxiety and distress on waking from sleep.
- Wide-awake and full of energy when it is time to go bed.
- Fear of falling asleep through conviction that she will not wake again.
- Starts as about to fall asleep.
- Adversely affected by touch and noise.
- Chatters constantly.

Fever
- Temperature is very volatile with constant fluctuations between heat and cold, or a constant sensation of waves of heat flowing through the body.
- Constant thirst for cool drinks and heavy sweating.

Head
- Headache after sleep which often affects the left side.
- Pains are eased by lying down, warmth, or nasal discharge.
- Headache may be brought on by exposure to direct sunlight.

Eyes
- Sensitive and painful eyes which itch, sting and feel worse for being touched. Nevertheless, child rubs them constantly in search of relief.

Ears
- Ear pain (often left-sided, or moves from left to right) with accompanying sore throat.

Nose and Throat
- Blocked nose in the morning with sneezing.
- Nose feels easier after a nose bleed.
- Hoarseness in the morning with sharp pain or tickling in throat that leads to a choking sensation.
- Unpleasant sensations in throat are made worse by empty swallowing and better from swallowing food. Cool drinks are soothing while warm ones make things worse.
- Throat is very sensitive to touch so that a tight collar around the neck causes distress.
- Sore throats are often left-sided or begin on the left and move to the right.

Digestion
- Bloating which is relieved by passing a stool.
- Difficulty passing stools because of throbbing pains in rectum.

Worse from
Heat
Warm rooms
Draughts
Touch
At night
Waking from sleep

Better for
Fresh, cool air
Cold drinks
Onset of discharges
Eating
Movement

Ledum

Mental Picture
- Cross, withdrawn and irritable.

Fever
- Violent thirst for cold water.
- Although generally chilly, finds warmth of bed unbearable and throws off covers in an effort to cool down.

Head
- Pressing pain with headache that is relieved by fresh air and made worse by covering.

General features
- Hard, painful swellings with tearing pains.
- Pains move rapidly from site to site, and often move in a upward direction.
- Whole body feels bruised and aching.
- Joints are swollen and hot to the touch, but do not look red.
- Pains are generally much worse from warmth and better for cold applications or bathing.

Skin
- Itchy eruptions are worse on covered parts of the body and react badly to warmth of the bed, but feel better for cool air. Crusty eruptions around nose and mouth.

Worse from
Warmth in general
Being too heavily dressed
At night
Walking

Better for
Cold in general
Cool air
Bathing in cold water
Resting

Lycopodium

Mental Picture
- Gets very anxious before an event, but when it arrives feels fine.
- Dislikes being alone and needs the reassurance of someone around, even if it is in an adjacent room.
- Fears the dark, ghosts and strangers.
- Child goes into extreme tantrums if corrected or ticked off: can be very resentful.
- Hurried in movements and tends to get words jumbled up because of speaking too quickly.
- Sensitive to noise, music and pain: dislikes being hemmed in or having restrictive clothing around the neck.

Fever
- Although chilly, dislikes being kept too warm or having rooms too stuffy and airless.
- Once sweating has occurred, feels very thirsty.
- Likely to experience sudden flushes of heat.

Head

- Crushing headaches that are made worse by warmth, getting over heated and lying down.
- Head pains are eased by cool, fresh air, and gentle moving about.

Eyes

- Chronic tendency to develop styes with very sticky, pussy discharges.

Ears

- Ear pain with thick, offensive-smelling, yellow discharge which often affects the right side.
- Noises in ear or deafness with sensation as though hot liquid were flowing in ears.

Nose and Throat

- Tendencies to develop one cold after another with sinus problems and very blocked nose.
- Catarrh may be thick and yellowy-green in colour with tendency to settle at the back of the throat.
- Ulcerated throat which feels better for warm, and worse for cold drinks.
- Choking and burning sensations in throat.

Chest

- Coughing causes a severe headache and feels worse for taking a deep breath or for swallowing saliva.

Digestion

- Burning sensations in stomach are better from warm drinks and worse from cold.

- Discomfort in stomach comes on immediately after eating.
- Digestive uneasiness often comes on from 'nerves' before an exam or a stressful event. This results in lots of rumbling, gurgling, diarrhoea and butterflies in the stomach.
- Abdomen is so uncomfortable that pressure of clothes is very unpleasant: waistbands need to be loosened.

Sleep
- Wakes from sleep in a bad temper, but feels brighter once up and about.

Skin
- Terrific dryness and irritability of the skin causing burning pains and violent itching which are much worse for warmth of the bed and soothed by contact with cool things. Eruptions may weep a bloody or watery discharge.

Worse from
Warm, stuffy air or warm applications
Cold draughts
Weight of bedclothes
Over-tiredness
On waking
Touch
In the afternoons and early evening

Better for
Warm drinks
Moderate warmth
Loosening clothes
Open air

Uncovering
Gentle exercise

Mag phos

Mental Picture
- Tearful and complaining, but not inclined to violent tantrums or outbursts of anger.
- Listless, lethargic and very unwilling to do anything that involves effort.
- Forgetful with general difficulty concentrating.

Head
- Throbbing headache with red face which feels better for firm pressure and fresh air.
- Facial neuralgia may be made worse by touch, at night and early morning. Discomfort is eased by warm applications.

Eyes
- Right eye more often affected than the left. Pain is felt in the socket and there may be accompanying spasms in the muscles of the face.

Nose and Throat
- Constant need to swallow even though it makes throat pain worse.

Chest
- Red face with coughing spasms which make it impossible to lie down at night.
- Talking, walking, and being exposed to a warm

atmosphere for an extended length of time make the coughing worse.

Digestion
- Sore mouth which makes eating difficult.
- Upset stomachs and toothache are made worse by cold drinks and better from warmth.
- Colicky, radiating pains with lots of wind that make infant bend double or press hands into painful area in search of relief.
- Infants with colic lie on back with knees drawn up, screaming with pain.

Worse for
Cold in any form
Touch
At night
Movement

Better for
Warmth
Rubbing
Bending double
Resting
Pressure

Mercurius

Mental Picture
- Very restless and fearful for no obvious reason: cannot keep in one position for long.
- Most distressed and agitated at night.
- Very hurried and flustered or completely indifferent.

Fever
- Alternating hot flushes and cold chills with shivering.
- Thirst is extreme with heavy and offensive-smelling sweating at night.
- Insomniac at night, although very drowsy during the day.

Head
- Whole head is sensitive with headache which is worse at night and on waking, and better when up and about. Pain may affect the left side more than the right.

Eyes
- Discomfort in eyes is aggravated by heat. Feels worse at night.

Ears
- Earache is especially distressing at night and may be accompanied by sharp pains and an offensive looking and smelling discharge.

Nose and Throat
- Raw, sore nostrils with thick, green, nasty-smelling discharge.
- Swallowing is difficult from dry, sore throat, but is constantly necessary because of increased amount of saliva.

Chest
- Coughing spasms make child feel very sick, and are worse on lying down, especially at night.

Digestion

- Nasty, sweet, metallic taste in mouth with increased amount of saliva.
- Tongue feels and looks swollen and flabby: takes imprint of teeth.
- Mouth ulcers may accompany general feeling of unwellness.
- Colicky pains and vomiting are made worse by bending forwards.
- Burning, watery diarrhoea may be worse as evening goes on.

Sleep

- Terrible insomnia from anxiety, restlessness and general discomfort. Sweating is particularly bad at night and may smell offensive. All symptoms are much worse at night.

Worse from

Extremes of either hot or cold
Cold draughts
At night and in the evening
In bed
Touch
Eating
Sweating
Lying on the right side

Better for

Moderate temperatures
Resting

Nat mur

Mental Picture

- Moves from one extreme of mood to the other: very sad or laughing and joking.
- May show contrary emotions: laughs in a sad situation, or becomes very weepy in a happy one.
- Child rejects any form of consolation and sympathy when distressed, just wants to be left alone to get on with it.
- If upset, cries in private or may bottle up anger and resentment.
- Very sensitive to noise in general, and specifically to music.

Head

- Giddy and sick from travelling: may also develop a headache.
- Head pains may also be brought on from delayed meal times: child looks pale with pain.
- Headache is much worse for movement, and child will have to lie down and sleep it off.

Eyes

- Gritty and dry sensations in eyes which tend to water easily: especially from walking in strong winds.

Nose and Throat

- Recurrent colds or allergic reactions which start with repeated sneezing attacks.
- Nasal discharge is abundant and clear: often feels as though a tap has been turned on.

- Nose runs excessively when bending forward: child uses endless paper tissues.
- Very runny nose which alternates with dry, blocked feeling with discharge that looks like egg white. Hoarse throat with tickling, irritated sensation.

Digestion
- Mouth and lips are noticeably dry: there may be a characteristic crack in the middle or on the corners of mouth.
- Tendency to repeated outbreaks of cold sores around mouth and nose which are brought on by emotional stress, colds or exposure to sunlight.
- Child wants foods with a strong savoury taste, especially salty things.
- Constipation may be troublesome with tremendous straining to pass dry, hard stools.

Skin
- Child is very sensitive to sunlight, often suffering problems such as prickly heat or hiving; headaches also may be brought on by over-exposure to the sun.
- Skin is generally dry with tendencies to crack easily, especially during the winter months.

Worse from
Extreme temperatures
Sunlight and hot weather
Stuffy rooms
Exercise
Touch or pressure
Emotional stress

Better for
Cold bathing
Open air
Fasting
Gentle movement

Nux vomica

Children often require this remedy after over-indulging in food or having too great a mixture of incompatible dishes. In other words, it is often the remedy required when a child is sick after a birthday party, provided the symptoms agree. It is also well indicated for symptoms which can follow a course of conventional medication such as constipation or general digestive upsets.

Mental Picture
- Very irritable, touchy and easily provoked.
- Easily frustrated and made to feel discontented.
- Picks quarrels with and is aggressive towards other children.
- Child reacts very badly to being ticked off or corrected, also does not respond well to sympathy or consolation.
- Very sensitive on both mental and physical levels, with general difficulty sleeping.

Fever
- Very chilly and irritable when feverish with marked dislike of exposure to cold in any form. Although child may look red and boiling hot, she or he cannot stand draughts of cold air and demands to be well covered.

Head

- Constricting pains that are better for napping.
- Sick headaches with constipation and total lack of appetite.
- Headache feels better for warmth and firm pressure.

Eyes

- Severe sensitivity to light on waking with profuse watering.
- Burning, smarting and itching of the eyes.

Nose and Throat

- Cold symptoms are worse indoors and better in the fresh air.
- Nose feels either blocked and dry or runs like a tap.
- Lots of sneezing with rawness of the throat.
- Pain in throat shoots to the ears when swallowing.

Chest

- Tickling, irritating, dry cough which is worse at night.
- Warm drinks give relief to coughing spasms.
- Very severe headaches accompany coughing bouts.

Digestion

- Toothache is brought on by exposure to cold air or chill and is relieved by warmth.
- Nausea with difficulty in vomiting: however, once it occurs, it relieves straight away.
- Wind and colicky pains that are made worse by eating, or pressure, and better for warmth.
- Constipation with lots of straining and urging, but stool seems to slip back into rectum rather than being expelled.

Worse from
Cold in general, especially draughts of air
Mornings
Disturbed sleep
Eating

Better for
Uninterrupted sleep
Lying down and resting
As the day goes on
Wet weather

Phosphorus

Mental Picture
- Mentally and physically easily exhausted.
- Child needs a lot of attention and reassurance and reacts well to it.
- Anxious and full of fears: of the dark, thunder, solitude and illness.
- Craves sympathy and cuddles.
- Very sensitive to all sorts of stimuli: light, noise, music, touch and odours

Fever
- Sudden alterations in circulation causing chilliness with flushes of heat.
- Although experiencing burning sensations, child may complain of icy-cold feet and legs.
- Burning thirst for ice-cold drinks which may be vomited back once warmed by the stomach.

Head

- Headache feels worse for warm, stuffy rooms and lying down. It is relieved by exposure to cool air, sitting up and eating a little.
- Child's face looks flushed and hot with headache.

Nose and Throat

- Very dry inside the nostrils with blocked feeling.
- Nasal discharge is often yellowy-green and nasty smelling.
- Colds readily go down to the throat and chest, often involving glands in the neck.
- The throat feels sensitive to touch and cold air, and there may be a constant need to cough in order to clear the throat.
- Painless hoarseness or loss of voice may occur.

Chest

- Hard, irritating, dry cough that feels worse for lying down and moving from one temperature to another.
- Feels more comfortable propped up in bed on a few pillows.
- Tight, constricted feeling in the chest which is relieved by warmth.
- Phlegm is usually yellow coloured.

Digestion

- Burning pains in the stomach that are relieved temporarily by cold drinks: warm food and drinks may cause vomiting.
- Nausea and vomiting are much worse in a warm, stuffy room.

- Diarrhoea may be painless and passed involuntarily: often worse in hot weather.
- Bowel movements may be preceded by colicky pains.

Worse from
Lying on the left side
Early evening
Darkness
Being alone
Excitement
Thunderstorms

Better for
Warmth
Eating
Uninterrupted sleep
Being massaged
Reassurance

Pulsatilla

Mental Picture
- Timid, weepy and in need of a lot of sympathy and attention.
- Moods can be changeable: moving from tearfulness to irritability or happiness very rapidly.
- Much better for a good cry, cuddles and consolation.
- May be very anxious and in need of reassurance.
- Child's cry is pathetic rather than irritable (as in Chamomilla or Nux vomica).

Fever
- Very chilly with a marked aversion to being in a warm or stuffy room.
- Although child's mouth is dry with fever, there is no thirst.
- Hot and cold flushes alternate with dislike of being kept too warmly-covered in bed.

Head
- Headache with upset stomach from overly rich or fatty foods.
- Pains get worse after eating and with the approach of evening.
- Relief is provided by firm pressure and cool applications. Gentle movement in fresh air also helps.

Eyes
- Conjunctivitis with thick, yellow discharge that causes the eyelids to stick together on waking.
- Eyes itch and burn with a constant desire to rub them for relief.
- Frequent styes with a tendency to affect the lower lid.

Ears
- Pains which are brought on by exposure to cold winds.
- Discharge may be thick and yellow or creamy-coloured with an offensive smell.
- Ears feel painful and blocked.

Nose and Throat
- Constant catarrh which is thick, yellowy-green and bland.
- The nose may feel sore and swollen.

- Blocked feeling alternates from nostril to nostril: it improves in fresh air, and gets worse indoors (especially in stuffy rooms).
- Child complains of loss of taste and smell with a heavy cold.
- Dry, sore throat with no thirst.

Chest
- Dry cough in the morning which becomes loose and more productive at night.
- Chest feels uncomfortable on lying down and forces child to sit up to breathe more easily.
- Phlegm which is coughed up is yellowy-green.

Digestion
- Nasty taste in the mouth with dryness, but no thirst.
- Heavily-coated tongue with white or yellow fur.
- Vomiting may occur after over-excitement or emotional upset.
- When feeling sick child complains of a horrible chilly sensation, but feels worse for a stuffy room.
- Burning sensation in stomach is worse for warm food or drink, and better for cool.
- Burning, violent diarrhoea which is worse at night and may be caused by eating too much fruit or ice-cream.

Sleep
- Child is sleepy on going to bed but is woken by becoming over heated during the night. Throws off bed covers in sleep, gets too cold, and pulls them back up again. Often sleeps with hands above the head, and pushes feet out of the covers because they are burning hot.

Skin
- Terrible itching which is made worse by contact with heat in any form, and relieved by cool air or washing.

Worse from
Warmth
Stuffy rooms
Heavy bedcovers
Humidity
Resting
Evening and night

Better for
Fresh, cool, open air
Gentle exercise
Cool food, drinks, washing and applications
Sympathy and attention
Firm pressure

Rhus tox

Mental Picture
- Extreme mental and physical restlessness which is especially marked at night.
- Sadness with weepiness over things that would not normally cause an upset.
- Child constantly moves about in search of a comfortable position.
- Withdrawn, lethargic and cannot be bothered with anything.

Fever
- Feverish to the point of delirium: may mutter in fitful sleep. Thirst may be unquenchable for cold drinks, especially at night. Very sweaty and trembly with feverishness which is intensified by taking warm drinks.

Head
- Severe headache which is relieved by warmth and bending the head backwards.
- Pains may be brought on by frustration or anger.

Eyes
- Styes with generalised swelling of the lids and profuse watering of the eyes.
- Eyeballs may feel sore with stiff feeling in eyelids.

Nose and Throat
- Sneezing and easy nose bleeds on waking.
- Hoarseness on beginning to speak which improves as voice is used.

Chest
- Dry, tickling cough that is brought on by exposure to the smallest draught of cold air.
- Raw feeling in air passages generally with bloody or salty taste in mouth.
- Coughing leads to severe headache.

Digestion
- Dry, sore, cracked lips and mouth with possible development of cold sores.
- Sore tongue with inflamed triangular tip.

- Strong colicky pains are relieved by moving about and bending double.
- Exhausted with involuntary passage of stools.
- Severe morning diarrhoea that is painless.

Sleep
- Very restless sleep, especially after midnight. Exhausting dreams that leave child worn out on waking.
- Yawns constantly because of exhaustion.
- Moves constantly about the bed in search of a comfortable position.

Skin
- Puffy skin eruptions that itch and burn intolerably. Skin feels more inflamed and uncomfortable in bed at night, with constant desire to scratch, which does not help.

Worse from
Cold, wet weather
Resting
Lying
Standing still
Initial movement
Second half of the night

Better for
Warmth
Warm bathing
Heat locally applied
Warm, dry weather
Wrapping up warmly
Continued movement

Ruta

Thirs is a remedy which has a particular affinity for symptoms that suggest injury to the periosteum (the membraneous sheath that covers bones). Pains that respond well to Ruta are bruised sensations which lead to a feeling of weakness in the area affected. The injured area is very sensitive to touch and may, or may not, be swollen. Pains are worse from resting, cold, wet and when lying down on the painful area or walking out of doors. They are better for warmth and moving about indoors.

Ruta may be indicated for injuries and bruises that initially responded well to Arnica, but that refused to resolve themselves completely. This is often the case with deep bruising that has affected the bones.

Sulphur

Although often indicated for symptoms involving irritation of the skin, because of its extremely dynamic and deep-acting nature, this is a remedy that should be used very sparingly and with caution. Do not repeat it frequently over a long period of time.

Mental Picture
- Very irritable, touchy and sorry for her or himself.
- Child can get to the point where it feels impossible to deal with him because of impatience and tantrums followed by sulking.
- There is a strong aversion to washing and a desire to avoid it whenever, and wherever, possible.

- Child lacks 'grit' or staying power with regard to things that need long-term stamina or persistence.

Fever

- Although very hot and disliking rooms which are over heated, cold draughts are not tolerated either.
- The head might feel uncomfortably hot while the feet are cold, or the feet can feel burning hot.
- Very thirsty for lots of drinks of water, but does not sweat.

Head

- Head pains are worse out of doors or when stooping and better for resting in a moderate temperature.
- Weekend headaches are common after the end of the school week.

Eyes

- Burning, itching and redness of the eyes.
- Eyelids may be very red around the margins with a yellowish discharge which dries into crusts.

Nose and Throat

- Recurrent colds with thick, offensive, persistent nasal discharge.
- Nose is stuffed up indoors and runs when outside.
- Child complains of discomfort in the throat like a sensation of a ball or lump which refuses to be moved on swallowing.

Chest

- Tightness and pressure in the chest which feels worse at night: child demands to have windows open for fresh air.

Digestion

- Definite dislike of fat, eggs and milk.
- Early morning, painless diarrhoea which causes child to rush to the toilet as soon as he or she is up.
- Red, sore, burning anus with diarrhoea.
- Alternation of constipation with diarrhoea.

Sleep

- Wakes regularly around 3 a.m. and finds it impossible to go back to sleep.
- Jerks violently as about to drop off to sleep.
- Child wants to sleep in: very difficult to rouse in the morning.

Skin

- Very unhealthy, itchy, inflamed skin which leads to a constant need to scratch. This is often so intense that it results in the skin weeping and bleeding.
- Skin generally feels worse for contact with warmth in any form, heat of the bed or washing.
- Child's skin may also react badly to woollen garments.

Worse from

Heat and warmth
Warmth of bed
Washing
After eating
Waking
Mid-morning

Better for
Dry, moderate weather
Lying on the right side

Veratrum album

Mental Picture
- Restlessness alternating with prostration and exhaustion.
- Symptoms may follow a shock from injury or a fright.
- Although withdrawn and quiet, child does not want to be left alone.
- Child may become frantic with discomfort.

Fever
- Very chilly, clammy and pale with shivering.
- Sweating is very marked and thirst is unquenchable for cold water.
- State of complete collapse with illness.

Nose and Throat
- Nose feels freezing cold with blocked sensation on one side.
- Frequent and violent sneezing.

Chest
- Cough is loose and rattling, but child has great difficulty raising phlegm.
- Belching accompanies the cough.
- Child presses against the stomach when coughing.
- Cough is made worse by breathing cold air or being in a warm room.

Digestion
- Lots of saliva in mouth with vomiting and diarrhoea which are both very severe.
- Terrible nausea sets in before vomiting and there may be colicky pains and cramping.
- Immediately during and after vomiting and diarrhoea child looks deathly pale and sweaty: sweats are especially marked on forehead.
- Diarrhoea may follow eating too much fruit.

Sleep
- Although prostrated, child cannot sleep from nausea and general discomfort.

Worse from
Cold and damp
Movement
Touch and pressure
Warmth
Passing a stool
Perspiration
At night

Better for
Resting
Lying down
Coolness

HOMOEOPATHIC REMEDIES AND THEIR ABBREVIATIONS

Remedy	Abbreviated name
Aconitum napelus	Aconite
Allium cepa	
Antimonium crudum	Ant crud
Antimonium tartaricum	Ant tart
Apis mellifica	Apis
Arnica montana	Arnica
Arsenicum album	Arsenicum alb
Belladonna	
Bryonia alba	Bryonia
Calcarea carbonica	Calc carb
Calcarea phosphorica	Calc phos
Calendula officinalis	Calendula
Cantharis	
Carbo vegetablilis	Carbo veg
Chamomilla	
Colocythis	
Cuprum metallicum	Cuprum
Dulcamara	
Eupatorium perfoliatum	Eupatorium

Euphrasia
Ferrum metallicum   Ferrum met
Ferrum phosphoricum   Ferrum phos
Gelsemium sempervirens   Gelsemium
Hepar sulphuris calcareum Hepar sulph
Hypericum perfoliatum   Hypericum
Ignatia amara   Ignatia
Ipecacuana   Ipecac
Kali bichromium   Kali bich
Kali carbonicum   Kali carb
Kali muriaticum   Kali mur
Kreosotum
Lachesis
Ledum palustre   Ledum
Lycopodium
Magnesia phosphorica   Mag phos
Mercurius solubilis   Mercurius
Natrum muriaticum   Nat mur
Nux vomica
Phosphorus
Phytolacca decandra   Phytolacca
Podophyllum
Pulsatilla nigricans   Pulsatilla
Pyrogenium   Pyrogen
Rhus toxicodendron   Rhus tox
Rumex crispus   Rumex
Ruta graveolens   Ruta
Sanguinaria
Silica
Spongia tosta   Spongia
Sulphur

Symphytum officinale	Symphytum
Thuja occidentalis	Thuja
Urtica urens	Urtica
Veratrum album	Veratrum alb

FURTHER READING

General introductory guides to homoeopathy, first-aid, and books on self-help

The Complete Homoeopathy Handbook: A Guide to Everyday Health Care, Miranda Castro, Macmillan, 1990

Everybody's Guide to Homoeopathic Medicines: Taking Care of Yourself and Your Family with Safe and Effective Remedies, Dr Stephen Cummings and Dana Ullman, Gollancz, 1986

The Family Guide to Homoeopathy: The Safe Form of Medicine for the Future, Dr Andrew Lockie, Elm Tree Books, 1989

How to Use Homoeopathy Effectively, Dr Christopher Hammond, Element, 1991

Homoeopathic Medicine at Home, Maesimund Panos and Jane Heimlich, Corgi 1980

Safe and Sound: The Complete Guide to First Aid and Emergency Treatment for Children and Young Adults, Linda Wolfe, Hodder and Stoughton, 1993

Homoeopathy, Medicine for the 21st Century, Dana Ullman, Thorsons, 1989

Homoeopathy, Medicine for the New Man, George Vithoulkas, Thorsons, 1985

The Complete Book of Homoeopathy, Michael Weiner and Kathleen Goss, Bantam, 1982

Homoeopathy: Headway Lifeguides, Beth MacEoin, Hodder & Stoughton, 1992

Homoeopathy and Children

Homoeopathy for Mother and Baby: pregnancy, birth and the post-natal year, Miranda Castro, Macmillan, 1992

Homoeopathy and Your Child, Lyle W Morgan, Healing Arts Press, 1992

Homoeopathic Medicine for Children and Infants, Dana Ullman, Piatkus, 1994

For a more in-depth account of a restricted number of homoeopathic remedies see *The Homoeopathic Treatment of Children: Pediatric Constitutional Types*, Paul Herscu, North Atlantic Books, 1991

Information on Vaccination

The Immunization Decision: A Guide for Parents, Randall Neustaedter, North Atlantic Books, 1990

Vaccination and Immunization: Dangers, Delusions and Alternatives, Leon Chaitow, C W Daniel, 1987

Nature's Child: guide, nourish and protect your child the gentle way, Leslie Kenton, Ebury Press, 1993

Articles

'The Immunisation Debate', *Childright*, January/February 1992

USEFUL ADDRESSES

Council for Complementary and Alternative Medicine
179 Gloucester Place
London NW1 6DX
Tel: 071 724 9103

Institute for Complementary Medicine
Unit 4
Tavern Quay
Rope Street
Rotherhithe
London SE16
Tel: 071 237 5165

Natural Medicines Society
Edith Lewis House
Ilkeston
Derbyshire DE7 8EJ
Tel: 0602 329454
(a charity representing consumer interests in alternative
medicine)

British Complementary Medical Association
St Charles' Hosital
Exmoor Street
London W10 6DZ
Tel: 081 964 1206

The Society of Homoeopaths
2 Artizan Road
Northampton
NN1 4HU
Tel: 0604 21400
(provides a register of professional homoeopaths with a
minimum of four years' training in homoeopathy)

The British Homoeopathic Association
27a Devonshire Street
London WC1N 3HZ
Tel: 071 935 2163
(provides a register of orthodox doctors who have undergone
additional training in homoeopathy)

The Hahnemann Society
2 Powis Place
Great Ormond Street
London WC1N 1RJ

The Informed Parent
29 Greyhound Road
Sutton
Surrey
SM1 4BY
(provides information on immunisation)

Ainsworths Homoeopathic Pharmacy
38 New Cavendish Street
London
W1M 7LH
Tel: 071 935 5330 (Daytime) 071 487 5252 (24 hour
answering machine service)

Helios Homoeopathic Pharmacy
97 Camden Road
Tunbridge Wells
Kent TN1 2QP
Tel: 8092 536393

Nelson's Pharmacies Ltd
73 Duke Street
London
NW1M 6BY
Tel: 071 629 3118
(licensed manufacturer)

Waleda (UK) Ltd
Hearst Road
Ilkeston
Derbyshire
DE7 8DR
Tel: 0602 303151
(licensed manufacturer)

The Homoeopathic Supply Company
4 Nelson Road
Sherringham
Norfolk
NR26 8BU
Tel: 0263 824683
(provides boxes for storing remedies, phials and other
homoeopathic supplies)

INDEX